Reimagining Aid

Studies of the Walter H. Shorenstein Asia-Pacific Research Center

Andrew G. Walder, Series Editor

The Walter H. Shorenstein Asia-Pacific Research Center (APARC) in the Freeman Spogli Institute for International Studies at Stanford University sponsors interdisciplinary research on the politics, economies, and societies of contemporary Asia. This monograph series features academic and policy-oriented research by Stanford faculty and other scholars associated with the Center.

Reimagining Aid

FOREIGN DONORS, WOMEN'S HEALTH,
AND NEW PATHS FOR DEVELOPMENT
IN CAMBODIA

Mary-Collier Wilks

Stanford University Press

Stanford, California

Stanford University Press
Stanford, California

Library of Congress Cataloging-in-Publication Data
Names: Wilks, Mary-Collier author
Title: Reimagining aid : foreign donors, women's health, and new paths for development in Cambodia / Mary-Collier Wilks.
Other titles: Studies of the Walter H. Shorenstein Asia-Pacific Research Center
Description: Stanford, California : Stanford University Press, 2026. | Series: Studies of the Walter H. Shorenstein Asia-Pacific Research Center | Includes bibliographical references and index
Identifiers: LCCN 2025027515 | ISBN 9781503643857 cloth | ISBN 9781503644809 paperback | ISBN 9781503644816 ebook
Subjects: LCSH: Women's health services—Cambodia | Medical assistance, American—Cambodia | Medical assistance, Japanese—Cambodia | Women in development—Cambodia | Non-governmental organizations—Cambodia | Public health—Cambodia—International cooperation
Classification: LCC RA564.85 .W55 2026 | DDC 362.109596—dc23/eng/20250925
LC record available at https://lccn.loc.gov/2025027515

Cover design: Ann Weinstock
Cover art: Wikimedia Commons, Danseuses Cambodgiennes: anciennes et modernes

The authorized representative in the EU for product safety and compliance is: Mare Nostrum Group B.V. | Mauritskade 21D | 1091 GC Amsterdam | The Netherlands | Email address: gpsr@mare-nostrum.co.uk | KVK chamber of commerce number: 96249943

Contents

Acknowledgments

Thank you first and foremost to the development workers who participated in this project. Your trust and openness made it possible for me to tell your stories.

I am deeply grateful for my excellent mentors, who enabled me to grow this project from an excited graduate student's spark of an idea to its final form. Thank you to Jennifer Bair for supporting this book from its earliest phase to the final read-through with her cutting insights and tireless editing. I also received invaluable guidance from Sarah Corse, Simone Polillo, Adam Slez, Sylvia Tidey, and Kiyoteru Tsutsui. This book also could not have come to fruition without the astute and supportive comments of my book workshop participants: Monika Krause, Joseph Harris, and Gowri Vijayakumar.

I appreciate my many colleagues and friends who have provided feedback to me through all stages of this research, particularly my chapter swappers Eliza Brown, Erin Michaels, and Isabel Pike. I am indebted to the participants of the Talks on Economy, Markets, Politics, and Organizations (TEMPO) workshop at the University of Virginia as well as the Gender Workshop and the Philanthropy and Civil Society (PACS) workshops at Stanford University. I am grateful to Andy Walder for his assistance with this project, my editor Dan LoPreto, the team at Stanford University Press, as well as my two reviewers who enabled me to deepen the contribution of this book. This project was also made possible due to generous funding from the America-Japan Society, the Center for Khmer Studies, the Department of Education's Foreign Language and Area Studies Fellowship, the Fulbright Institute of International Education, and the National Science Foundation.

I am profoundly thankful for my family, friends, and community who have shown up for the many challenges and successes throughout this project. I owe much to the love and constant support of my mother, Betsy Wilks, and my dog, Beignet, who slept on my feet or at my side for most this book's writing. I also would not be who I am without my mother's choice family of activists, scholars, and creatives who raised me to be curious about the social world. Additionally, I appreciate my graduate school colleagues, Pilar Plater-Nagao and Sarah Johnson-Palomaki, without whom graduate school, and the conception of this book project, would have been much less joyful.

I am grateful to Natalie Rupp for engaging in the never-ending, iterative conversational process that I needed to develop the ideas for this research as well as for accompanying me on my fieldwork journey. My fieldwork would not have been feasible without her love, support, and directional skills. This book is your accomplishment too. Finally, in the concluding stages of the project, I am thankful to Chase Gobble for his encouragement as well as his keen sense for all things design/creative. I am indebted to Chase, Adeline, and Eliot for showing me it was possible to start again. By providing me with the space to grieve, love, and feel safe, my scholarship has flourished once more.

Reimagining Aid

Introduction

In honor of International Women's Day, the United States Agency for International Development (USAID) hosts a workshop at the U.S. Embassy in Phnom Penh, Cambodia. At the event, a roundtable discussion takes place focusing on the question of why gender inequality persists in Cambodia and possible solutions. One Cambodian high school teacher poses the question—"How can we strive for women's empowerment and preserve our culture?" A Cambodian nongovernmental organization (NGO) director responds passionately, "What do you mean by culture? . . . if what you mean by culture is that we celebrate Khmer[i] New Year, bring food to the monks, wear special clothes, then that's nice." But, she goes on to exclaim, "Culture is often used to oppress women. We are not destroying Asian culture by women having more freedom. We need to have a dialogue about what is culture and how can women's equality be part of it." A Cambodian practitioner from a different NGO responds, "If we take up all these Western ideas about gender, how will we still be Cambodian? Asia needs to make its own way!" The panel presider tries to smooth over this debate, arguing it is important to speak out against problematic aspects of Cambodian culture while embracing others.

After the workshop, I sit outside with a Cambodian NGO worker, Sophy. Sophy is the head of the communications department at a U.S.-funded international NGO, U.S. Family Aid. Prior to taking that position, she worked for the U.S. Embassy for over ten years. She is a fluent English speaker and seasoned development worker. Sophy explains that she, of course, thinks it is essential for women to work, make money, and be inde-

1

pendent. "These are the good things about the Western way . . . otherwise, their husband can control them too much." Yet, as we talk, she tells me that she believes "the Japanese culture . . . and the other Asian donors . . . they are much closer to Cambodia's, you see . . . Americans are always trying to get women to speak out. I think the Japanese know you can make money, support your family, and maintain your values . . . this is the Asian way . . . the Western donors try to change too much."

Overhearing our conversation, a Cambodian NGO worker, Chantou, disagrees heartily. Chantou works for a local gender advocacy NGO. She responds to Sophy, stating, ". . . but the Japanese don't say anything about gender. Just as they don't say anything about the Cambodian elections![2] How can they help make change in our country for women? Their projects do not address this! Cambodian culture . . . there are many good things but there are many things that need to change." Sophy snaps back at her, "It is not the job of Western donors to change Cambodia."

In Cambodia, and around the world, the economic, political, and cultural influence of East Asian nations like South Korea, Japan, and China is rising. These changes are shifting the way that national development and ideas about what it means for women to advance in society are discussed in the Global South.[3] Cambodia is just one of many nations where Asian donors and aid organizations are playing a more prominent role in the development space. In the past, donors and international organizations based in the U.S., Europe, and Australia were the dominant actors in the production of prevailing global norms about what makes "good development" (Thornton, Dorius, and Swindle 2015). However, the increasing influence of East Asian donors is challenging Western hegemony around the world (Greenhill, Prizzon, and Rogerson 2016). Nongovernmental organization (NGO) practitioners, charged with implementing development in their countries, are particularly active in this discussion.

This book presents findings from a multisited ethnography, in which I conducted participant observation in multiple NGOs funded by the U.S. and Japan that implement projects aimed at upgrading women's health in Cambodia (Swidler and Watkins 2017). As we start to see in Chantou and Sophy's conversation above, I find that NGO practitioners in Cambodia perceive there to be two competing paths to national advancement for nations to follow, one "Asian" and the other "Western." Strategically employing these two competing models of development, Cambodians construct new visions of the role of the state, civil society, the market, and gender in national advancement, as well as the place of Cambodia in the world. This book examines what these competing imaginaries of Asia and the West might mean for the future of aid and development as practitioners in the Global South articulate new, alternative ways of understanding what it means to be "developed" and how to get there.

Moving Beyond the Global-Local Binary

In a moment of global transformation, it is necessary to reconsider "global" development norms and the way we study foreign aid. Historically, researchers assumed that international development organizations, at least formally, promulgate well-known global norms, such as the pursuit of gender equality or the promotion of neoliberalism. Studies of international actors investigate the construction of these "global" norms. Then, scholars investigate whether these norms are adopted, modified to fit the local contexts, or resisted on the ground in recipient nations through processes of "localization" or "vernacularization" (Boli and Thomas 1999; Bernal and Grewal 2014; Dromi 2016; Levitt and Merry 2009; McDonnell 2016; Mosse and Lewis 2006; Ong and Collier 2007).

Studying aid through the global-local lens has garnered numerous insights, yet it has become increasingly clear that "global" development norms have origins in a particular nation, typically one with the material resources to promote its development vision throughout the world. This means that "global norms privilege those of a particular 'local' and are better understood as globalized localisms" (Halliday and Carruthers 2009: 6). Developed nations in "the West" like the U.S., European countries, and Australia have long been considered synonymous with "the global." Yet, as the chapters of this book will demonstrate, the decline of Western dominance and the competing hegemonic efforts of Western and Asian donors break down the global-local binary as a useful tool for understanding aid. In Sophy and Chantou's debate we can start to see that practitioners use rhetoric that juxtaposes Asia and the West in the process of defining development on the ground.

However, this book does not aim to simply introduce a new binary, Asia-West, to studies of international development, but instead to illustrate that the emerging development norms of Asia and the West, respectively, contain a multiplicity of meanings that are continually reworked through the practices of development workers. Development work asks practitioners to envision the best path towards advancement for recipient nations within the changing global order. In doing so, development, not unlike nationalism, frequently requires practitioners to draw boundaries around their country in comparison to donor nations that aid them (Puri 2003). Practitioners engage what I call "development imaginaries": a complex set of beliefs about development that are not fixed. Imaginaries are employed in ways that are both change-oriented and status-quo oriented. For instance, Cambodian practitioners use rhetoric about "the Asian way" to contest the American donor practice of pushing mothers into the labor market without addressing childcare needs. In contrast, other Cambodian practitioners draw on notions of "Asian tradition" to justify not engaging in advocacy for reproductive rights. Consequently, the purpose of this project is to interrogate the binaries we typically use to produce knowledge about development, such as local/global, state/civil society, traditional/modern, and now West/Asia. I illustrate that these binary frameworks are put into use in a multiplicity of ways by development practitioners and explore the consequences of this for recipient nations and foreign aid (Alexander 2006).

Studying Development in Aid Chains

To move past the global-local framework, we must investigate the "contact zones" in which development practitioners remake aid in encounters between the global, regional, national, and local scales (Grewal 1996; Puri 2003). As nonprofit organizations that provide information, services, or advocacy aiming to advance or "develop" nations in the Global South, NGOs are one such contact zone. NGOs are typically funded by donors in the Global North while the provision of services takes place in the Global South. Many scholars have examined global-local interactions, providing qualitative studies of the localization of global policies in NGOs in recipient nations and quantitative analyses of the diffusion of global policies and their impacts on government policies and/or public opinion around the world, as well as research into the ways localization of policies can come to influence global policies (Bernal and Grewal 2014; Pierotti 2013; Rinaldo 2013; Tsutsui 2018).

To rethink our conception of "global" development norms without falling into essentializing a new macroregional Asia-West binary, we need a method for studying international development that can uncover both the origin location of globalized localisms, account for emerging regional norms, trace how norms are modified as they are put into practice, and investigate how new norms—development imaginaries—come to challenge the global. We need a transnational method that recognizes that development is "constituted through interactions between multiple locales" (Radhakrishnan 2011: 18; Radhakrishnan 2022).

Studies of global commodity chains, which trace how products are designed, produced, and sold across the world, provide a transnational method that examines how things are constituted through interactions across various locations (Benzecry 2022; Tsing 2021). Treating aid projects as a cultural product to be traced, I undertook a multisited ethnography of the multiple organizations that comprise two transnational "aid chains" (Swidler and Watkins 2017; Wilks, Richardson, and Bair 2021). Aid chains contain donor organizations that provide funding for aid projects in developing nations. In my case Japan's and the U.S.'s bilateral agencies, which provide funding from the governments of Japan and the U.S. to Cambodia, are the donor agencies. The next links in these aid chains are the international NGOs (INGOs) these donors fund, which maintain their headquarters in developed nations. Headquarter offices were maintained in Tokyo and Washington, D.C., in the aid chains studied here. INGO headquarters offices then manage INGO country offices in recipient nations, like Cambodia. Finally, INGOs typically implement development projects via support to local partners, such as local NGOs or government organizations in the receiving country.

Through an in-depth study of two aid chains, this book analyzes the multiple scales at which development is constructed and made into a reality. I analyze how development norms are made into organizational practices through everyday interactions between donors, NGO practitioners, and recipient stakeholders. The transnational aid chain framework allows me to analyze how development practitioners work across multiple organizations and scales as they engage incoming ideas from the regional, national, and community levels, imagining new meanings in the process. In doing so, this book provides both an opportunity for us to rethink gender, development, and foreign aid in a moment of global transition as well as offering a new method of studying development as it is produced at multiple moments in aid chains. However, before outlining my findings, I analyze how the shifts in the global power balance this book investigates came to be.

International Development and a Changing Global Order

When asked about international development, most people list topics like these: Poverty reduction. Capitalist growth. International human rights. Democracy promotion. Gender equality. This is because international development organizations frequently work together to determine and disseminate dominant development norms and policies (Cold-Ravnkilde, Engberg-Pedersen, and Fejerskov 2018; Swiss 2018). To do so, organizations such as the United Nations and the World Bank work together with donor agencies, like USAID, as well as a wide variety of INGOs in international meetings and networks. One World Bank report defines global norms as "standards of expected behavior about how things ought to be conducted and are deemed crucial for society to flourish" (Martinsson 2011). Such norms are often codified into policies, like the UN's Sustainable Development Goals, and prescribe what "good development" looks like.

The legacy of wealthier countries prescribing the best path for advancement to other nations can be traced back to colonization. Specifically, during the second era of European colonial expansion (approx. 1840–1914), European nations colonized huge portions of the world, particularly in Asia and Africa. Alongside transformations in social beliefs, colonization required nations in the Global South to reorganize their economies to serve the metropole (McMichael and Weber 2021; Puri 2003). Colonizing nations believed reorganizing economic and cultural values in the colonies would "modernize" what colonizers considered "backwards" or "traditional" societies, particularly the "poor" and "native" women of these nations (Chen 2010; Grewal 1996; White 2023). The importation of European ideas about what makes a nation modern to the colonies can be considered an early iteration of the global diffusion of ideas on how nations should advance—that is, development norms.

Yet, the story of foreign aid as we know it today begins after decolonization and the Second World War. Between 1945 and 1960, dozens of new states in Africa and Asia gained independence (McMichael and Weber 2021). Due to losses from the Second World War and decolonization, European power declined, enabling the U.S. to emerge as a new global leader (Inkenberry 2005; Mann 2003; Meyer 2010). In the late 1940s, the U.S. established what we now know as foreign aid by providing funding to Europe for rehabilitation with the intention of reestablishing the global economy. Shortly after, during the Cold War, U.S. aid increased primarily to what was then called the Third World, emphasizing capitalism and democracy in opposition to the Soviet Union, priorities which have had a lasting impact on today's global development norms. Furthermore, in the 1940s and 1950s, the U.S. gained clout within two major development institutions, the World Bank and the International Monetary Fund, which would give it lasting influence over global development norms (Lancaster 2007; McMichael and Weber 2021).

When the world faced a global debt crisis in the late 1970s and early 1980s, the U.S. and the U.K. pushed for market-based economic measures or "neoliberal" policies to become the globally dominant paradigm for development (Babb and Kentikelenis 2021; Fourcade-Gourinchas and Babb 2002). The World Bank and International Monetary Fund assisted in this project, employing rhetorical commitment to neoliberalism as well as coercive mechanisms, like structural adjustment loans, which required nations in the Global South to enact market-based reforms to gain access to development loans (Ganti 2014). Hence, due to its position in the world order at these historic moments, the U.S. has played a prominent role in defining development since the 1940s (McMichael and Weber 2021). Thus, while the mechanisms of development intervention have transformed since colonization, European and American governments as well as multilateral organizations still envision needy nations in the Global South requiring assistance to develop (Escobar 1995). Western donors have long provided much-needed funding to local stakeholders in the Global South, but only for projects stakeholders in the U.S. and Europe believe to be deserving of support.

However, currently, we are living through another moment of geopolitical transition, shifting the nature of foreign aid and the development sector. "The post–Cold War order, which deemed that 'Western liberal democracy and free-market capitalism held all the answers,' has been destroyed, wrote Roger Cohen, the *New York Times* Paris bureau chief in the days prior to the World Economic Forum's 2023 meeting in Davos" (Radhakrishnan and Solari 2023: 149). Several events in the early 2000s began to sow doubt about the U.S.'s place in the world order. These events include, first, the 2001 terrorist attacks and their aftermath and, second, the 2008 financial crisis (Arrighi 2009; Inkenberry 2005). The World Economic Forum now predicts that by 2030, the U.S. will no longer be the dominant economic power in the world.

In contrast, in the beginning of the twenty-first century, new models of economic development were on the rise in Asia. Japan and South Korea, hailed for their rapid economic ascent, emerged as prominent examples of successful developmental states (Chu 2016). Many Asian nations, such as Singapore and South Korea, weathered the 2008 financial crisis better than their Western counterparts. China is rapidly becoming a global economic powerhouse and an increasingly important player in international geopolitics, challenging the U.S.'s post–Cold War monopoly on global power (Ciccantell and Bunker 2004). It is now hotly debated if China or India might become the next global hegemon or if the world is moving towards a more multipolar global order (Arrighi 2009; Ciccantell and Bunker 2005; Inkenberry 2014; Radhakrishnan and Solari 2023; Songchuan and Shulong 2011).

Whatever the outcome of these larger geopolitical shifts, powerful Asian nations have produced alternative models of social and economic development, such as the well-known "developmental state" in which the government is in the driver's seat of economic development (Chorev 2020; Chu 2016). While Japan, South Korea, and China differ from each other in their approach to development assistance, these countries are increasingly juxtaposing their foreign aid priorities against those of the West (Stallings and Kim 2017). Such models provide a counterpoint to the dominant "global" development norms produced by the U.S. and other Western nations, enabling people in the Global South to consider multiple paths to development.

Regional Transformations and Donor Gender Regimes

The donors in this study display both national and regional differences in their aid. Investigating national variation in donor practices is indispensable for understanding the construction of regional development models. Research provides increasing evidence for the importance of variations in aid between donors from different nations (Stallings and Kim 2017; Stroup 2012; Wilks 2019). For instance, a foreign aid donor's nation of origin shapes whether that donor provides direct funding to a recipient government or supplies aid through the private sector or civil society[4] organizations (third sector, nongovernment, noncorporate organizations, like churches or NGOs). For example, Germany provides a large amount of direct aid to the governments of recipient states, although it funds civil society organizations as well. In comparison, the U.S. bilateral agency that distributes aid funds, USAID, prides itself on its preference for supporting civil society organizations and the private sector (Dietrich 2021).

Consequently, the original focus of this project was mainly on national variation in aid donors. Wanting to contribute to our understanding of differences among donor countries, in 2016 I set out to study the impact of variation in donor priorities on gender and development projects in Cambodia (Wilks 2019). Yet what I found was that, while there are clear differences between donors from every *nation*, Cambodian practitioners drew on distinctive donor patterns to construct what I came to see as *regional* development norms. This is because, although there is national-level variation between the aid projects provided by different donor nations in both East Asia and the West, Cambodian practitioners see broad similarities in the practices of donor nations from the two regions.

For instance, in general, nations in the West are more likely to fund civil society organizations than those from East Asia. In contrast, East Asian donors are more likely to direct funding towards the state and provide more loans than grants (Stallings and Kim 2017). Similarities between the aid models of Western nations are due to the fact that these countries developed their foreign aid models during the 1950s and 1960s, using one another for reference. They have continued to be highly engaged in the global development space, attending the same conferences and other convenings, and shaping their aid programming accordingly (Lancaster 2007). In contrast, China and South Korea, newer donors, report using Japan's aid as a reference point when they developed their aid programs. This inter-Asian referencing in the development of foreign aid programs leads to key similarities in the aid models of East Asian donors as well (Stallings and Kim 2017).

Consequently, this book analyzes how, alongside knowledge of geopolitical transformations, Cambodian practitioners utilize donor differences to construct regional development imaginaries. I chose to analyze INGOs, and donors based in the U.S., because of that country's role as the historic hegemon and its dominant role in the construction of global development norms described above. I compare the U.S. case to INGOs and donors from Japan. Japan was selected because it is historically a regional leader in Asia. As the first East Asian nation to industrialize, Japanese foreign policy has long pushed the notion that Japan is a leader in Asia (Black 2017).

Beginning in the mid-1950s, Japan paid reparations to four countries in Southeast Asia—Myanmar, the Philippines, Indonesia, and Vietnam. Soon after, Japan began to offer government-to-government assistance in the form of loans, small grants, and technical assistance to numerous Southeast Asian nations (Er 2013). By the late 1980s, Japan was the first East Asian nation to fund NGOs and social development projects (Black 2017; Rei-mann 2010; Stallings and Kim 2017).

Japan was also the first East Asian nation to articulate and lobby for an "East Asian" development model to challenge the Washington Consensus in the 1980s (Taniguchi and Babb 2009). Finally, if one positions East Asian donor countries on a continuum vis-à-vis their Western counterparts, Japan represents an intermediate case. South Korea adheres more strictly to the norms of the Organization for Economic Cooperation and Development (OECD) Development Assistance Committee while China, as a non-OECD member, has a more distinctive foreign aid model (Stallings and Kim 2017).[5] This makes Japan a key player that development actors draw on in describing the Asian development model.

The book illustrates how Cambodian practitioners integrate the national differences of development organizations from Japan and the U.S. into regional development imaginaries. Specifically, I investigate a women's health project funded by each nation. Gender and healthcare are key sites of contestation about the role of men and women in national advancement (Puri 2003). In each chapter, I examine different aspects of the U.S. and Japan's own *donor gender regimes*, or the ways in which donor projects are embedded within and diffuse their own nation's dominant gendered beliefs through distinctive interventions into Cambodia's state, civil society, and private sector (Atlani-Duault 2007; Connell 1990).

As we will see in subsequent chapters, while Japanese and American donors are committed to improving women's health in Cambodia, they want to do so in different ways. In the eyes of American donors, the market is primary, with the state and civil society filling in only as necessary. The general idea is that women's advancement will come from their having equal access to the market. These priorities lead to support for INGO projects that improve private and nonprofit reproductive and maternal healthcare. Japanese donors, on the other hand, emphasize state capacity, which they see as a necessary force directing the market. In this model, women deserve access to public healthcare as citizens and fertility is encouraged. This results in Japanese-focused INGO projects that support the public sector and are narrower in scope, as the focus is on upgrading maternal health services as opposed to supporting women's health more generally.

Yet, development norms and donor priorities do not transfer uncontested into recipient nations but are instead rejected, co-opted, and modified in varying ways as they are put into practice in different countries (Bernal and

Grewal 2014; Vijayakumar 2021). Cambodian practitioners interpret the gender regimes of the U.S. and Japan through the lens of regional development imaginaries as they resist and remake donor projects. In the next section, I examine why Cambodia is a key case for investigating the way development is being reimagined in the Global South.

The Increasing Power of "Asia" in Cambodia

Cambodia is a small country with a history of strategically maneuvering between larger powers. Before being ousted in 1970, Prince Sihanouk led Cambodia through the Cold War and garnered resources for the country by carefully balancing Russian, Chinese, and U.S. interests (Osborne 1994). Today, the prime minister must balance the rivalry between China and the U.S. (Pich and Aun 2023). Cambodians have also been negotiating foreign aid and INGO interventions in their country for over thirty years. During the 1970s and 1980s, Cambodia was ruled by the violent Khmer Rouge regime and then faced over a decade of civil war. In 1991, the United Nations Transitional Authority in Cambodia (UNTAC) supported the formation of a new government, fair elections, and economic liberalization in Cambodia (Hughes and Un 2011). During the UNTAC era, abundant international funding opportunities attracted INGOs from around the world to Cambodia and supported the founding of multiple local NGOs (Hughes 2007; Un 2005). For many years, Cambodia could be considered a "donor darling" with one of the highest concentrations of nongovernmental organizations (NGOs) in the world (Frewer 2013).

Throughout the 1990s, international organizations played an essential role in developing ministry policies, ensuring democratic elections, and providing needed social services in the war-torn nation. In 2010, development assistance still made up 61 percent of the nation's budget. Bilateral donor agencies from the U.S., Europe, and Australia as well as INGOs largely funded by those nations held, at least in the UNTAC era and the following decade, substantial authority in the Cambodian context. Although the percentage of the national budget comprised of international aid has decreased, falling to approximately 28 percent in 2018, development organizations are still deeply embedded in the Cambodian government and in the everyday life of Cambodians (Open Development Cambodia 2018).

Nevertheless, the current political context in Cambodia differs for Western versus East Asian donors. International NGOs with funding from the U.S., Europe, and Australia face an increasingly complex political land-scape. Starting in the late 1990s, a single political party, the Cambodian People's Party (CPP), has consolidated power. As part of this consolidation, the CPP has been progressively restricting NGOs that promote human rights, democracy, and collective action. While this is a challenge for all NGOs, the degree to which it affects different NGOs varies. Many U.S.-funded INGOs have faced political repression, and a few have been asked to leave the country. Even those U.S. INGOs that successfully partner with the Cambodian government must be careful to maintain government ap-proval to continue operating.

Two additional forces have lessened Western influence in Cambodia. First, the World Bank categorized Cambodia as a lower-middle-income nation in 2015, instead of as a lower-income nation. This pushed aid donors to direct funding to more needy countries. Second, in 2017, the CPP out-lawed the main opposition party, the Cambodian National Rescue Party, ensuring a CPP victory in the 2018 national election. Donors from the United States and Europe, which have long provided the bulk of funding to Cambodia's NGO sector, are now committing fewer resources in light of these political and economic developments. The CPP also accused the U.S. of colluding with the Cambodian National Rescue Party, increasing tension in Cambodia-U.S. relations.

In contrast, East Asian nations, including Japan, South Korea, and China, have maintained or grown their influence in Southeast Asia. When Western organizations responded to what they saw as a deterioration in the political environment, Prime Minister Hun Sen claimed that the U.S. and the EU could cut aid, since the government has secured promises from China to replace that money, largely through loans (Thul 2017). Addition-ally, consistent with the fourth plank in Cambodia's National Development Plan, the Cambodian government is now emphasizing regional integration and intra-Asia relations. Cambodia's Foreign Direct Investment (FDI) is also dominated by Asian investors (UNCTAD 2020). In 2019, Cambodia received 3.7 billion U.S. dollars in Foreign Direct Investment, and 73 per-cent of investors were from Asian nations (UNCTAD 2020).

Specific to the donors this book investigates, USAID and Japan's bi-lateral Japan International Cooperation Agency (JICA) both started pro-viding development aid to Cambodia at the same time during the UN transitional era. In Cambodia today, Japanese policymakers and develop-ment officials promote the rhetoric of the rise of Asia with NGOs like the

Asian Friendship Society; they promote the idea that Japan is a leader in Asian development in response to China's active attempts to provide an alternative framework to Western development or "an Asian development model." Japan competes with China to have a leadership role in Cambodia (Hughes 2009).

Outside of aid, Japan, South Korea, and China's economic development as well as cultural products are seen as models to emulate in Cambodia and many other Southeast Asian nations (Hoang, Cobb, and Lei 2017). For instance, young Khmer adults, especially those in urban areas, follow East Asia beauty trends carefully. South Korean looks are the most referenced beauty ideal, but Japanese fashion is also popular. Khmer young adults often get haircuts like their favorite K-pop stars, buy Korean skin lightening products, or shop at stores carrying Korean and Japanese fashion. One INGO worker tells me, "Maybe twenty years ago people wanted to look like Americans, but now it's all about South Korea and Japan." The growing power of East Asian nations in Cambodia has a significant impact on the way that Cambodians think about economic, political, and social development possibilities in their nation (Nam 2011).

Defining the Development Imaginaries

Living and working in this context, Cambodian development workers are in a broker role, navigating so-called "global" norms, regional changes, demands of foreign aid donors, and their nation's own context. Development, or what it means for a nation to advance, is itself a discursive formation that imagines an intervention to improve, which is always being contested and reformed (Li 2005). In their broker role, NGO workers combine incoming ideas from the global, regional, national, and local scales to make development meaningful in practice, employing the two dominant development imaginaries about Asia and the West.

Charles Taylor (2004) defines a social imaginary as "the ways people imagine their social existence, how they fit together with others, how things go on between them and their fellows, the expectations that are normally met, and the deeper normative notions and images that underlie these expectations" (23). Similarly, a development imaginary holds multiple schemas about the advancement of citizens and a nation, such as interpretations of the role of the state in development or what it means to advance women in society. A development imaginary can be defined as the schemas, or "sets of cognitive associations, developed over repeated experience, that present information and facilitate interpretation and action," that people employ to imagine the paths to progress their nation (Hunzaker and Valentino 2019: 950). It includes an inherent comparison of how that path compares to other nations, and the types of social values that accompany different paths to development.

Cambodian practitioners' "Asian" and "Western" development imaginaries are not the first cultural narrative to gloss over national differences to make claims about what makes a modern "Asian" nation or to use ideas about Asia to destabilize Western claims to universal knowledge about modernity, capitalism, or development. In the late nineteenth century, a debate raged about the nature of Eastern versus Western civilizations. Leaders in China, Japan, and India all articulated different notions of Eastern civilization to differentiate Asian nations from those of the imperializing West (Jenco 2013). In a recent example, in the 1980s and 1990s, "Asian values" language was employed by political leaders in Southeast and East Asia. Singaporean Prime Minister Lee Kwan Yew is known for stating that Asia was the new center of the world (Barr 2002; Ojendal and Antlov 1998). Such rhetoric was used to explain the economic success of strong states in many Asian nations, to challenge the idea that liberal, Western values are universal, and, sometimes, to justify authoritarianism (Ojendal and Antlov 1998; Sen 2017).

Yet, these usages of "Asian values" often employ many of the problematic binary frameworks noted earlier in this chapter, such as traditional/modern or state/civil society. Asian values rhetoric frequently homogenized the cultural, geographic, and political diversity of Asia into a singular set of, largely Chinese, values. Nevertheless, citizens in Asian nations did find regional sentiments about the rise of Asia compelling, and this continues today. As Chen (2010) explains, "the globalization of capital has generated economic and cultural regionalization, which has in turn brought about the rise of Asia as a pervasive structure of sentiment. As a result, both a historical condition and an emotional basis exist for new imaginings of Asia to emerge" (214).

Asian studies scholars now try to capture the "new imaginings of Asia" and their consequences, documenting diverse interregional comparisons and Pan-Asian rhetoric (Hoang 2015). Instead of reifying a particular value system, scholars push for the need to investigate how different Asian traditions travel, how they can be used as comparative models or new reference points, and how they are hybridized in practice (Chen 2010; Hoang, Cobb, and Lei 2017). Inter-Asian referencing scholarship acknowledges that ideas and practices from the West, such as capitalism, have impacted Asian nations and identities. At the same time, these ideas have been modified, localized, and contested in Asian nations, enabling new inter-Asian forms to emerge. Consequently, we must keep a careful eye on the fact that what is considered "modern Asia" is constantly evolving and hybridizing (Chen 2010).

Thus, my study of development imaginaries takes up the call of inter-Asian referencing scholars by investigating the multiplicity of surprising ways practitioners use the two development imaginaries, sometimes explicitly juxtaposing them or borrowing from one to challenge the other. Cambodian practitioners draw development imaginaries to navigate work and define what they think would advance Cambodia in various settings (Swidler 1986). Such schemas are not fixed, singular, reified imaginaries of Asia and the West, but frequently reworked, contested, and employed strategically in diverse ways by Cambodian practitioners.

In practice, I frequently saw Khmer practitioners employ development imaginaries in three major ways. First, sometimes practitioners will *reinforce* the need to enact donor practices through assumptions about Asian and Western models. For instance, when Japanese INGOs support the Cambodian state's capacity, Cambodians describe such programming as "the Asian way" of doing development and argue that this practice works "for our peoples." Here, practitioners draw on similarities between Asian nations to reinforce project activities that meet their approval and to implement them.

Second, Cambodian practitioners will use the Asian versus Western models to directly *reject* the practices of donors or foreign managers in their organization. For example, even though Japanese managers want to consider integrating a discussion of birth control methods and birth spacing into their INGO's programming, Khmer practitioners argue those topics are too difficult to discuss within "Asian" cultural and political traditions. They contend only "Western" NGOs discuss political topics like family planning, and then those organizations get blacklisted by the Cambodian government.

In contrast to uses where national differences are erased to emphasize regional similarity, Khmer practitioners will sometimes parse out differences between nations in Asia or the West to reject the practices of their donor. In doing so, they argue that a different donor nation's practices are ideal or problematic, compared to their donor. In the U.S.-based INGO, when one American manager thinks their INGO should lobby local officials, Cambodian practitioners bring up Scandinavian-funded organizations, which are known to be more advocacy-oriented, in comparison to the softer approaches of U.S.-funded INGOs. They warn foreign practitioners that many Scandinavian organizations are blacklisted, advocating that the softer U.S. model is the ideal way of the West. This illustrates the complex usage of national and regional rhetoric, which sometimes universalizes "Asia" or the "West" while at other times parsing out national differences between donor practices when it suits practitioner purposes.

Third, the imaginaries are sometimes used to *hybridize* practices and modify donor gender regimes. As we will see in chapter 4, at the U.S.-based INGO, practitioners contend that U.S. practices around gender equality in the workplace do not account for the unique challenges mothers face. Instead, they argue for a hybridization of Asian and Western gendered beliefs to provide needed supports for new mothers. Each of these three uses of development imaginaries—reinforce, reject, or hybridize, as well as their consequences for the practice of international development—will be analyzed in subsequent chapters.

Cambodia is not the only nation where citizens may be rethinking development within our changing global geopolitical context (Balogun 2020). China, Japan, and South Korea provide generous foreign aid funding to many South and Southeast Asian nations (Stallings and Kim 2017). East Asian nations are also increasingly supporting numerous aid projects in Africa (Sibiri 2019). Thus, the ways in which Cambodians use competing "Asian" and "Western" development imaginaries to interpret aid may well shed light on the changing nature of international development and the possibility that new norms are being produced in Asia and around the world. A world where development is understood through competing models of Asia and the West is one that will come to provincialize understandings of "global" development norms to their origin point in the West.

Gender and Race in Development Imaginaries

Gender and race are key sites for sense-making and contestation about what it means for a nation to be advanced (Fernandes 2017; Grewal and Kaplan 2002; Heng 2018; Hoang 2015; Radhakrishnan 2011). First, Cambodian practitioners must make sense of incoming beliefs about gender within their own cultural context. Ideas about gender relations, motherhood, and femininity are often deeply bound up in conceptions of national advancement or gender regimes that donors export (Connell 1990). This is particularly true of women's health projects that aim to advance maternal health and family planning needs. Some of the most contentious cultural debates in the U.S., such as abortion, bring up disagreements about the meaning of motherhood and women's role in the home and workforce (Luker 1985). These domestic debates impact foreign aid. For instance, the Mexico City Policy was implemented by President Reagan in 1984 and required INGOs to agree to neither perform nor actively promote abortion as a method of family planning in other nations as a condition for receiving federal funding. For decades, the U.S. ended and restarted foreign aid funding for abortions depending on the political party in power. Donors export gendered assumptions from their own nations when supporting development projects.

Development practitioners implementing women's health projects also encounter gendered beliefs from the global and regional levels. Transnational advocacy groups promote dominant global norms and policies for promoting gender equality around the world, like the UN's Committee on the Elimination of Discrimination against Women (CEDAW) Treaty or the UN's Sustainable Development Goal Five, which aims to achieve gender equality and empower women and girls. Gender norms also travel throughout Asia when it comes to ideals of masculinity and femininity. For instance, Japan borrowed the phrase "good wife, wise mother," from feudal China to describe an ideal Asian woman's role in society. The phrase was endorsed by the Japanese government during World War II to promote nationalism and women's supporting role in the growing economy (Fengxian 2012; Fujimura-Fanselow 2014). Similarly, today, many Cambodians import and explicitly emulate South Korean forms of femininity.

Cambodia also maintains its own cultural understandings about what it means to be a "good" woman or man in society, and these understandings do not remain stagnant over time. Legend has it that the original ruler of Cambodia was an unmarried woman, Soma. Historical analysis shows Cambodian women were treated with relatively similar respect to men of the same class status for most of Cambodia's history, as the social class hierarchy was the predominant differentiating force in Cambodian society. Dominant patriarchal conceptions of gender difference that remain influential today were imported to Cambodia with a more patriarchal brand of Hinduism in the ninth century. Such conceptions really took off in the nineteenth century, due to the influence of the Thai court on the Cambodian king in the 1820 and 1830s, and French colonization, which began in the 1860s (Jacobsen 2008).

From 1900 into the 1960s, gender differences and the lesser position of women in society were further bolstered by nationalist conceptions of women and men during Cambodia's anticolonial movement and post–French liberation nation-state building. Today, when Cambodian political leaders and some of the participants in this study talk about a return to "traditional" Cambodian values that assume men have higher status than women, they are looking selectively at the writings and lifestyles of elites in the nineteenth and twentieth centuries, instead of the gender relations of everyday Cambodians for most of Cambodia's history (Jacobsen 2008).

When it comes to gender inequities today, Cambodia is ranked 102 out of 146 countries on the 2024 Global Gender Gap Index, which assesses countries on measures of gender parity in economic participation and opportunities, educational attainment, health and survival, and political empowerment (Pal et al. 2024).[6] Women in Cambodia are underrepresented in leadership positions both in the political system and the workforce. In 2023, only 16 out of 123 members of the national parliament were women (Vicheika 2023).

Cambodia does have a strong history of both men and women in the workforce, with the International Labour Organization (ILO) reporting the country has the highest female labor force participation rate in East Asia and the Pacific region. Eighty percent of women in Cambodia work in comparison to 90 percent of men. However, women are more likely than men to engage in microbusinesses, low-wage work, or nonwage work than men (Gavalyugova and Cunningham 2020; USAID 2016). This is due to strong cultural norms around family that expect men to be breadwinners and women to be less visible in the public eye while bearing most of the burden in caring for the home and children. These dominant expectations mean women in Cambodian today are more likely to work in informal employment where they can combine work-family demands, such as subsistence farming or selling a service from their home (Gavalyugova and Cunningham 2020).

While these data paint a general picture of gender inequalities in Cambodia, the experiences of Cambodian women vary and are shaped by intersecting identities, such as geographic location, age, and socioeconomic status. For example, the gendered experiences of young, unmarried women working in factories around Phnom Penh are very different from those of rural, Cham women, a Muslim minority group that largely lives in rural provinces. All cultures, including Cambodia's, hold within them multiple ideas about what it means to be a woman or man of that nation and a diversity of gendered experiences (Radhakrishnan 2011).

International and local NGOs addressing women's development, and later gender and development, began popping up in Cambodia as early as 1993. In response to the different gender inequalities the country faces, the forms of gender advocacy NGOs engage in vary greatly. For example, there are NGOs that work with labor unions and female garment workers to mobilize for better wages. There are also many international NGOs in Cambodia that try to "mainstream" gender equality into their programming, but identify themselves as working in a specific sector, like health or agriculture, such as the American INGO in this study. There are also numerous urban NGOs that define their mission as challenging inequalities between men and women in work, politics, and the household. Specifically, implementing aid projects in women's health, like those in this study, brings up a recipient nation's cultural beliefs about the roles of men and women in work and family, regulation of women's sexuality, and the meaning of mothering (Connell 2012; Klausen 2015).

Consequently, the development organizations in this study that advance women's health are a key space where practitioners draw on numerous ideas from domestic norms, donor priorities, regional references, and international advocacy to define the place of men and women in the advancement of Cambodia. Cambodian practitioners frequently employ the imaginaries of Asian and Western development to deliberate between this multiplicity of gender beliefs as they implement development projects in their nation. It is important to note that when practitioners draw on beliefs about gender there is sometimes slippage between levels. For instance, practitioners often intertwine ideas about Asian-ness and Cambodian-ness. We see this in Sophy and Chantou's debate at the beginning of this chapter when the two women argue about whether USAID's gender equality programming undermines or can be integrated into Cambodian or "Asian" culture.

Additionally, as we will see throughout the chapters, as practitioners define and contest the path for Cambodia's development, the Asia/West imaginaries are often intertwined with rhetoric about Cambodia's family "traditions" and what it means to be an appropriately "modern" woman or man. Such debates also go back to the colonial era in which colonizing countries often portrayed colonized women as "victims" of backwards cultural traditions. In contrast, during the struggle for independence, nationalist groups often portrayed gender norms as essential to their nation's sacred and long-standing traditions (Narayan 1997). Women's roles in society and family structures continue to be at "the heart of dilemmas of modernity and tradition in a nation" (Puri 2003: 137).

Second, development imaginaries and their regional comparisons involve not just gender but also assumptions about race in the global order. Racial identities are created by society and assign unequal social meanings to different groups of people, often based on skin tone. These identities are built on comparisons between groups of people and are frequently reinforced by powerful social institutions (Alexander 2006; Heng 2018). Yet, the remaking of racial identities and hierarchies is often done in response to historical moments that provide enough ambiguity around power relations for new ideas about race to emerge (Heng 2018). The economic and political challenge Asian nations are posing to U.S. influence has provided such a moment (Hoang 2015).

Development imaginaries are employed by practitioners to challenge the racialized power dynamics inherent in the international development sector, in which the majority of countries that are the "most" developed, wealthy, and models for national advancement are predominantly comprised of and governed by white people. People of European descent have long dominated knowledge production about development because the U.S. and European nations have been the leading aid donors and purveyors of global development models since colonization. These models have inherently assumed white peoples to be "modern" and racialized others to be uncivilized or backwards (White 2023).

Development imaginaries enable inter-Asian and regional comparisons which Cambodian practitioners use to articulate a new racial order. Asianness and economically developed nations like South Korea and Japan are contrasted to Western others, challenging the assumption that white citizens of Western nations and their cultural values are inherently at the top of the development hierarchy that has predominated since colonization. International development organizations are not the only site where people are contesting the dominance of knowledge produced in predominately white, industrialized nations. For instance, in a study of the global cosmetic surgery industry, Menon (2023) finds South Korean, Singaporean, and Malaysian surgeons promote an "Asian" approach to cosmetic surgery. They promote an Asian aesthetic at international conferences to decenter Western medical approaches. Similarly, the leaders of nations like China, Japan, and India increasingly promote Asian models of development. This book investigates microlevel processes through which Cambodian practitioners decenter Western and white knowledge about development.

Cambodia and the Global South

By analyzing Cambodian actors' role in reimagining development, this book tells a new story about Cambodia. Cambodia has been subject to what Fahlberg (2023) calls "epistemic disequilibrium," or "a drastic imbalance in the types of narratives produced about a community or population which, in their totality, create an inaccurate or incomplete image of a place or people" (16). In modern times, Cambodia has long been associated with the violent Khmer Rouge regime. This genocide did unthinkable damage to Cambodian peoples, who live with generational trauma to this day. Nevertheless, in the rest of the world, the Khmer Rouge is often the only thing many people know about Cambodia. Such a story is used too often to paint Cambodia, and Cambodians, as impoverished victims. These types of stories are told too often about nations in the Global South (Escobar 1995).

This book offers a story about Cambodians that paints them in a new light. With their long history negotiating the demands of international donors, Cambodian development practitioners are agentic and intentional in their work and personal lives. They make sense of new incoming beliefs, combining them into new imaginations of what it would mean to advance themselves and their own nation. The competing development imaginaries they have constructed are contributing directly to the global process of foreign aid regionalization. These practitioners should have a place in how Cambodia is represented to the rest of the world.

Data Collection

To conduct my in-depth study of transnational aid chains, I undertook multiple research trips to Cambodia between 2016 and 2024. During the 2018–19 academic year, I was based in Cambodia where I carried out approximately 12 months of continuous fieldwork. In this time, I undertook a multisited ethnography, observing within the multiple organizations that make up two aid chains. I spent five months in a Japanese INGO's office in Cambodia. I give this organization the pseudonym Japan Services Asia (JSA). I observed program implementation, staff interactions with visiting headquarters staff, and JSA's work with its local implementing partner, the Provincial Health Department of Steung Treng.[7] Next, I spent four and a half months in the Cambodian office of a U.S.-based INGO, which I call U.S. Family Aid (USFA). During this time, I also observed USFA's cooperation with its government partner, the Cambodian Center for Health Communication. After that, I conducted two and a half months of ethnographic observation in a local NGO that implements USFA's programming, which I gave the name Cambodian Development Society (CDS).

Additionally, between spring 2018 and fall 2019, I conducted three months of research in Washington, D.C. This included short-term observations at USFA's headquarters and 16 in-depth interviews with INGO staff based there. Three interviewees worked at USFA while the remainder were employed by other Washington, D.C.-based INGOs implementing health and gender programming in Cambodia. I also conducted interviews with two employees of USAID in Washington, D.C. Finally, to get a general sense of the rhetoric in the U.S. development sector, I attended eleven international development conferences and workshops in Washington, D.C., in which USFA staff were in attendance or speaking.

In 2019, I spent three months in Tokyo. There, I conducted short-term observation at the headquarters office of Japan Services Asia. I also conducted 18 interviews with staff in Japanese INGOs, and 4 of those interviewees worked for JSA. Additionally, I interviewed 2 staff from the Japanese bilateral agency, JICA, and 1 from Japan's Ministry of Foreign Affairs in Tokyo. I also attended eight international development events in Tokyo to better understand the development sector. Figure 1 provides a simple representation of the two aid chains in this study.

In Cambodia, I also supplemented my ethnographic data via in-depth interviews with development practitioners in INGOs, local NGOs, bilateral donors, and multilateral agencies that have programs in the areas of gender and health. I conducted 135 interviews in total. These interviews took place during preliminary data collection in the summers of 2016 and 2017, during the 2018–19 academic year, and during two follow-up visits to Cambodia in 2023 and 2024. Using a semi-structured interview guide, I inquired about the personal and professional histories of practitioners, their role in the INGO or NGO, and their goals for the intended beneficiaries of

FIGURE I. The Japanese and U.S. Aid Chains.

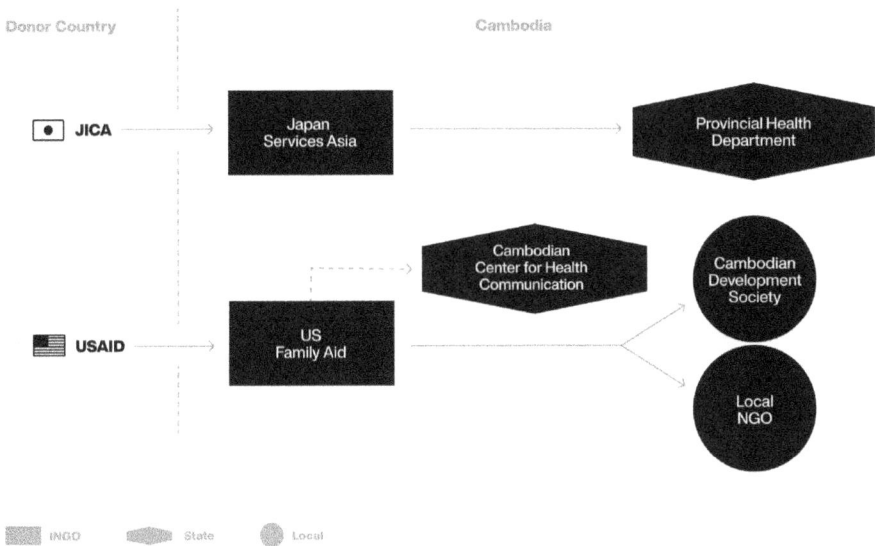

Donor Country   Cambodia

| JICA → | Japan Services Asia | → | Provincial Health Department |

| | | Cambodian Center for Health Communication | Cambodian Development Society |

| USAID → | US Family Aid | | Local NGO |

INGO   State   Local

their work as well as for themselves. This allowed me to gain a more general sense of the sector, where the INGOs in which I observed fit into it, and to follow up on program outcomes during my 2023 and 2024 research trips.

The INGOs in this study, Japan Services Asia (JSA) and U.S. Family Aid (USFA), were selected because each is funded by its nation's bilateral aid agency (JICA and USAID, respectively); both organizations have worked in Cambodia for over twenty years; and advancing women's health is a main goal for each organization. However, due to donor demands, each INGO had different ways of implementing women's health projects. USFA was implementing a 10 million U.S. dollar USAID health project over five years. Aside from its USAID project, USFA also implements numerous projects for other international donors from the U.S. and Europe in the areas of maternal health, family planning, and malaria prevention. This book examines USFA's largest project and its staff, a USAID project on "health behavior change," which aims to promote health behavior change across multiple interconnected health sectors including water, sanitation, and hygiene, maternal and child health and nutrition, family planning, and malaria in five different provinces across Cambodia.

To implement the project, USFA both partners with private clinics to upgrade and regulate the quality of their services and provides funding to

TABLE I. Interview Breakdown.

Organization	Number of Interviewees
Donor Country Context	
Japanese Donor Organizations	4 (2 orgs)
Tokyo-based INGO Headquarters	19 (16 orgs)
U.S. Donor Organizations	3 (1 org)
Washington, D.C.-based INGO Headquarters	16 (11 orgs)
Cambodian Context	
Japanese INGO Country Offices	27 (25 orgs)
U.S. INGO Country Offices	29 (25 orgs)
Local NGOs	30 (25 orgs)
Europe- or Australia-based INGOs or bilateral agencies	5 (5 orgs)
Korean donor office in Phnom Penh	2 (1 org)

local NGOs to provide health education. As local NGOs implement project activities on the ground, USFA practitioners spend most of their time monitoring and reporting. This is why, in addition to observing USFA staff in Phnom Penh, observing project implementation in the aid chain required I observe at the local NGO subgrantee, Cambodian Development Society. Per USAID's directive, USFA also partners with the national health subagency, the Cambodian Center for Health Communication, to help create a monitoring system for private and nonprofit health actors.

In contrast to USFA, Japan Services Asia (JSA) conducts a maternal and newborn health project with approximately 1 million U.S. dollars in JICA funding over a four-year period. JSA works only on one project in one province, Steung Treng. It maintains a few corporate donors and individual sponsors and those funds are used to conduct supplemental activities for the same project. JSA cooperates closely with the provincial health department to assist public health officials in implementing maternal and child health services. The organization does not implement any other projects or work with any other partner organizations, such as local NGOs. Since they do not subgrant to local NGOs to implement services, JSA has a small office in Phnom Penh where program managers work occasionally, but staff spend most of their time in JSA's provincial office in Steung Treng implementing project activities alongside public health officials. Because of these differences in aid chain configuration, my study of the Japanese-funded women's health project involved observation in only one organization in Cambodia as opposed to two.

As an ethnographer, I embedded myself into the everyday work life of each site as much as possible, completing whatever tasks NGO directors needed, including research projects, grant writing, searching for funding, editing documents, giving English lessons to staff, and assisting with hiring by reviewing applicants. In each INGO, I attended staff meetings on topics such as programming and planning, monitoring and evaluation, and budgeting. I also accompanied practitioners on field visits, observed workshops and trainings, and attended donor meetings. Moreover, after building rapport, I spent time with INGO staff outside of work hours, accompanying them to lunch, having after-work drinks, or attending family gatherings. These relationships allowed me to get a sense of how practitioners made sense of their careers, identities, and development more broadly. Because of the nature of this data and the fact that practitioners play a key role in the construction of competing development imaginaries, the book focuses mainly on development practitioners instead of beneficiaries.

This book finds its roots in my work as a grant writer and researcher at a local Cambodian NGO in 2011. The NGO where I worked implemented programs for women and children funded by diverse donor INGOs and foundations. Working there, I was struck by how differently donors from distinct nations defined gender empowerment and how local practitioners modified projects from different countries. It was through this experience that I began to think about the inequalities involved in the process of international aid; I saw how resources and ideas from all over the world flow through NGOs to affect the lives of all who encounter them.

Yet, despite this desire to study power inequalities in foreign aid, my own legibility as an American, white, cis woman holds inescapable power dynamics, which inevitably shaped my relationships with practitioners and stakeholders wherever I went. Conducting a multisited ethnography in three different nations required careful reflection about how my own positionality may shape data collection and modify my understanding of the data (DeVault 1996). First, my nationality, American, simply places limits on my knowledge of the full context of Cambodia or Japan. My position as an American also created power imbalances wherever I went, as most Cambodian practitioners associated me with Western donors. This meant many Cambodian workers initially spoke to me using the same rhetoric they do with foreign donors, and with deference. They also sometimes understood me as a promoter of the Western development model and its accompanying values.

Since I went back and forth to Cambodia several times between 2017 and 2024, over time I got to know Khmer workers well and spent informal time with them on weekends and evenings. This provided greater insight into their perspectives. It also allowed me to build their trust that I would not be reporting back to foreign staff or donors. Conversational Cambodian language skills were also essential, enabling me to examine differences in how workers speak, in English with donors and in Khmer with other workers. While my positionality necessarily shaped our interactions, sometimes it also did so in ways that provided me with insights I may not have otherwise had access to. Khmer staff would complain to me specifically in the hopes a foreigner might have more power to convince donors to change some practices, detailing how and why they needed to be modified for Cambodia. Or when several practitioners heard I was studying one "Asian" and one "Western" INGO, they would frequently offer their perspective on the different models. These responses to my project helped me become aware and begin to take note of the fact that Khmer practitioners were employing a regional development imaginary to comprehend their work, which eventually became the major topic of this book. My positionality and research methods are discussed in more detail in the methodological appendix.

Structure of the Argument

This book forges a new direction in the study of international development in a moment of geopolitical transition; it uses a novel method by studying development norms as they are produced at multiple moments in transnational aid chains. It illustrates the processes through which international development norms are changing and the key role of actors in the Global South in this process. To make this case, chapter 1 first defines foreign aid, INGOs, and women's health in the changing global context. Chapter 2 investigates the partnerships Japan Services Asia and U.S. Family Aid create with the Cambodian state. Chapter 3 examines how both donor gender regimes and the development imaginaries modify the women's health activities each INGO implements. Chapters 4 through 6 take an in-depth look inside the organizations, investigating the making of development in transnational workplaces. Chapter 4 investigates how workplace interactions result in different solutions to work-family conflicts in each INGO. Chapter 5 documents how INGO managers try to match donor financial practices to the logic of patronage and appropriate compensation in Cambodia.

Next, chapter 6 analyzes how Cambodian practitioners use the development imaginaries to construct differing career ambitions and professional identities, in ways that frequently do not perfectly align with donor intentions. Finally, the conclusion revisits Cambodia after the COVID-19 pandemic, and it also addresses the changes foreign aid is currently undergoing in our shifting geopolitical context. Then, by briefly investigating the development imaginaries in Vietnam and Ethiopia, I argue that practitioners in the Global South more broadly are playing a key role in reconstructing the power dynamics inherent in foreign aid. The conclusion goes on to consider what the development imaginaries may come to mean for the future of the global order, democracy, civil society, and gender equality.

Throughout these chapters, I illustrate that what flows along transnational aid chains is not just money and material aid but contending ideas about the role of the state, market, civil society, and gender in the development process. Donor gender regimes offer a partial explanation for why we see new understandings of development on the ground in Cambodia. This book takes seriously the role that practitioners at each link in the transnational aid chain play in making development into a reality. Development is not simply a question of whether local actors follow or resist global norms or donor demands. Rather, development in the current moment is about the diverse ways regional imaginaries are used to modify dominant understandings of what it means for nations to advance.

ONE

Transnational Feminism, Global Health, and the Changing Landscape of Foreign Aid

In the summer of 2011, I worked as an intern at a local NGO in Cambodia. Around six in the morning one day, my Cambodian coworker, Lakena, picks me up on her motorbike to head to the NGO's office in Kandal province, just outside Phnom Penh. We ride past the rapidly developing cityscape, bustling with people beginning their day, until the scenery changes to wooden houses and rice fields. As we arrive at the provincial office, the staff are hurrying to set up for a training, putting out chairs, hanging posters, and printing flyers. The NGO works with survivors of gender-based violence and women in poverty. Lakena informs me they will be giving a training on entrepreneurship and small business ownership this morning.

As an intern, I am not yet aware of the ubiquity of such trainings on the international development scene. I inquire why the staff selected that topic. Lakena laughs a little bit and explains, "it is *a way* of helping the women." She tells me entrepreneurship can help survivors to gain money and independence. However, pointing at me, an American, she asserts, "it is also *your* culture," as the training was funded by the NGO's U.S.-based donor. She reports that if an NGO wants to get funding, they must understand "the culture" of America, Europe, and Australia. But, she goes on to explain, if the women complete these trainings, we can give them small grants that they can use to start home businesses *and* provide food for their kids. The latter, although not necessarily sanctioned by the donor, was a big part of the reason NGO workers thought the trainings were useful. If they helped women set up small food carts with the grant, their families could also eat the dishes they sold.

In 2018, I returned to Phnom Penh and went back to visit this local NGO. As a coworker and I catch up, she tells me the donor landscape has changed since my internship in 2011. The organization still has funding from U.S. donors, but they are also working with Korean donors now. The Korean donor supports not entrepreneurship projects but maternal literacy. NGO workers go to the homes of mothers in rural areas and help them learn to read to their children. Softly, she tells me they also make a slight modification to this project. Despite donor directives, they include women who are not mothers in their trainings so those women can gain reading skills and eat the donor-provided lunch. The director tells me that when it comes to gaining funding, these days, they must negotiate "the culture" of East Asian donors as well.

Why do Lakena and other NGO workers understand themselves to be remaking development projects under the constraints of "the cultures" of foreign nations and regions? And why did the landscape for NGOs in Cambodia shift to include more East Asian donors between 2011 and 2018? Cambodia is just one nation where global transformations are altering foreign aid and international development, modifying the way projects to empower women and upgrade healthcare are implemented. For this reason, before investigating international development in the context of Cambodia, this first chapter looks at the history of and current transformations to foreign aid, NGOs, gender equality, and women's health programming globally.

Defining Foreign Aid and INGOs

Foreign aid refers to assistance that one country voluntarily transfers to another. It can take the form of a financial grant or loan as well as food, supplies, military assistance, knowledge transfer, or other types of humanitarian assistance (Lancaster 2007). Most donor nations maintain bilateral aid agencies, which are government agencies charged with dispersing foreign aid funding, like the United States Agency for International Development (USAID) or Japan International Cooperation Agency (JICA).

NGOs are nonprofit organizations that provide information, advocacy, and services aiming to advance or "develop" nations in the Global South. When engaging in advocacy, NGOs also raise issues, like environmentalism or reproductive rights, in international forums such as UN conferences, and mobilize local groups to pressure their governments (Ferree and Tripp, 2006). NGOs have also been enlisted in the provision of services like healthcare, education, and economic empowerment activities. International NGOs, or INGOs, like the two main organizations in this study, are NGOs headquartered in one nation (often in the Global North) that provide services in at least one other nation.

Starting in the post–World War II era, numerous changes to the foreign aid sector have set the stage for INGOs to play a key role in aid dispersal. Globally, since 1850, more than 25,000 INGOs have been founded (Boli and Thomas 1999). Like foreign aid, a number of INGOs originated to provide relief and assistance to victims of World War II in Europe. For instance, the Cooperative for American Remittances to Europe (later the E is changed to stand for "everywhere"), or CARE, is an INGO that was founded in 1945 to provide care packages to World War II survivors. When the UN was created in 1945, INGO participation was included in its charter. At this time, several nations also set up INGO committees to advise their government on relief work and humanitarian aid, with the U.S. starting such a committee in 1946 (Lancaster 2007).

As detailed in the introduction, foreign aid, which has its origins in the Cold War era, began with a focus on economic development and state-to-state assistance. However, by the early 1980s, there was a global push for foreign aid to broaden its focus, which had largely been on economic development, to include "soft" assistance like healthcare, education, and poverty relief (Lancaster 2007; Stroup 2012). This push coincided with the global promotion of neoliberal policies through structural adjustment loans in the 1980s. Enacting structural adjustment policies meant that states in the Global South often provided fewer public social services. INGOs came to be seen as ideal nonstate providers of soft aid, filling in the new gaps in social service provision. Assistance through NGOs, both local and international, was and continues to be promoted by the United Nations and the OECD's Official Development Committee (Reimann 2010).

In consequence, throughout the 1990s foreign aid donors increasingly provided funding for NGOs to deliver a portion of their development assistance. This led to the "NGO boom," with large numbers of local and international NGOs founded throughout the 1990s and early 2000s (Fechter 2019; Macdonald 1995; Packard 2016). Since then, NGOs have been prominent organizations in the international development sector. Specifically, as we will see below, NGOs provide the organizational form through which women's movements in many nations gained funding and international legitimacy. Women's advocacy, often through NGOs, made gender equality a global aid priority.

Gender and International Development

Transnational feminist advocacy made gender equality and activities that address it a core component of international development and foreign aid (Goetz 2020). Transnational feminism is the term used to discuss women's activism across borders (Desai 2015). Transnational feminist organizing brings women's groups from all over the world to engage in cross-border coalitions and debates. Throughout the second half of the twentieth century, women's movement groups and organizations played a key role in defining gender equality and women's empowerment as an essential component of development.

Transnational women's organizing has a history of successful advocacy campaigns as early as campaigns for temperance, education, and suffrage, starting in the 1800s. Early transnational organizing was dominated by women's groups from Western Europe and the U.S. For instance, the French Association Internationale des Femmes (International Association of Women) began in 1868, and the International Council of Women was founded in Washington, D.C., in 1888. Despite the dominance of women's groups from the West in transnational organizing, there is also a long history of women's groups in non-Western countries (Narayan 1997; Tripp 2006). China, Japan, India, Korea, and Burma all had their own large, active suffrage movements that joined Western organizers at international meetings. Not unlike debates we continue to see today, these early transnational feminists disputed the role of Western dominance in women's suffrage era organizing. For instance, Chilean feminists argued that European suffragists were too individualistic and had limited concern for the well-being of families (Tripp 2006).

After numerous nations passed laws giving women the right to vote, transnational women's advocacy declined in prominence in the early 1900s. Western feminists did continue to collaborate with women's groups in the Global South on issues like women's health or education. Yet the assistance of Western women's groups was often tied up with colonizing and "civilizing" missions. Starting in the 1940s, women's groups across the Global South increasingly allied with nationalist and anticolonial movements, which meant relationships with Western women's groups were often strained.[1] In this time period, many feminist movements in the Global South began, not due to Western feminist intervention but as part of anticolonial mobilization in their nations (Tripp 2006).

By the 1960s, colonization had ended or was in the process of ending in many nations in the Global South. Levels of mobilization were high around the world due to anticolonial and nationalist movements. Additionally, many European nations and the U.S. also had high rates of organizing at this time. In the U.S., the women's liberation movement was highly organized and active during the Civil Rights era. As women's movements began to make connections across borders, transnational women's organizing started to take off again.

In the late 1960s and early 1970s, women's groups from the West were again dominant players in what they called a "global" feminist movement. For instance, in the early 1970s, the term Women in Development was coined by a Washington-based network of development professionals. They argued that women in the Global South were not benefiting equally from the economic development paradigms promoted by aid actors throughout the 1950s and 1960s (Kanji and Pimbert 2003). Foreign aid donors did not take seriously women's role in a nation's economic development (Boserup 1970). Transnational feminist groups advocated for foreign aid donors to take up the Women in Development paradigm to address these problems, bringing the issue to international meetings.

By 1975, the first UN Conference on Women was held in Mexico City. Women's groups from all over the world came together alongside member states, private sector organizations, and unions. There it was decided the UN would have a "decade for women" and put in place sustained, long-term efforts to lessen gender inequities around the world (UN 2020). The UN then held Conferences on Women in 1975, 1980, 1985, and 1995, providing a site for transnational feminist groups, NGOs, churches, and unions to come together to discuss, debate, and advocate for women's issues throughout the decades (Keck and Sikkink 1999).

Yet, as the UN conferences and feminist transnational organizing took place throughout the last third of the twentieth century, there was a shift in North-South power dynamics. In 1938, the International Council of Women was made up of 78 percent affiliate councils based in Europe and the U.S. By 1963, it was only 47 percent affiliates from Europe and the U.S. (Goetz 2020). By the 1980 UN Conference on Women, held in Copenhagen, North-South tensions were at an all-time high as feminist groups from the Global South critiqued the Western-led transnational feminist movement. They argued that "global" feminism made homogenizing assumptions about women's needs without accounting for the ways differences in race, class, caste, ethnicity, religion, ability, and nationality shape women's advancement in society (McMichael and Weber 2021). Global feminist organizing was also critiqued because women's groups from the Global North often acted as if they had "made it" in relation to women in the Global South, who needed aid from the Global North. In making such claims, women in the Global North ignored inequalities that continued to plague their nations, such as women's limited political representation, the gender wage gap, or the fact that women continued to face household violence (Tripp 2006).

Feminists from the Global South also argued the global feminist movement was embedded in the liberal feminism of the U.S., which contended that economic and legal systems should be modified to benefit men and women equally. This meant mainstream Western feminism pushed for women to have power within the existing colonial legacies and capitalist system, instead of challenging the system as a whole (Das 2023). Living through the neoliberal restructuring of the 1980s, groups like DAWN (Development/Economics for/by Women), which originated in India in 1984, promoted discussions of the role of gender equality in the debt crisis and global poverty (Moghadam 2005). Feminists in the Global South argued that transnational feminist organizing should focus on collective mobilization that modified the global economic system, because issues of underdevelopment disproportionately impact women (Ferree and Tripp 2006; Kanji and Pimbert 2003; McMichael and Weber 2021).

By the 1985 UN Conference on Women in Nairobi, 60 percent of women's group attendees were from the Global South. In this moment, "the overall feminist center of gravity began to move from the North to the South" (Tripp 2006: 62). At this time, the Women in Development model, which did not adequately address the role men need to play in changing unequal family, political, and economic relations, was replaced with the Gender and Development, or GAD, model.[2] GAD was intended to switch the focus of development programs from "women" to the social relations, processes, and structures which gave rise to women's disadvantages. GAD attempts to address the differential impact of the global economic system on women and to account for women's different social identities (Kanji and

Pimbert 2003). Challenging Western dominance in transnational women's organizing, women's groups from the Global South were successful in adding new issues, like the flow of labor across borders, gender budgets, and gendered quotas in politics to the global agenda (Tripp 2006).

The final conference in Beijing, in 1995, is seen as the most important of the Conferences on Women. It brought together 17,000 participants, including 6,000 government delegates, more than 4,000 accredited NGO representatives, a host of international civil servants, and around 4,000 media representatives. At this conference, 189 countries unanimously adopted the Beijing Declaration and Platform for Action (UN 2020). The declaration set the future agenda in which nations committed to work towards women's empowerment and gender equality (Keck and Sikkink 1999; Tripp 2006). Additionally, transnational feminists were successful in getting numerous other global policies put in place at other international conferences, like the 1979 Convention on the Elimination of All Forms of Discrimination against Women, the 1996 International Labor Organization Convention on home workers, and the 1999 UN Jomtien Resolution on Education for All.

Gender equality was also integrated into the UN's Millennium Development Goals. These goals were meant to offer a development paradigm for governments and development organizations around the world. In the early 2000s, women's groups cooperating with the UN Human Rights Council also integrated rights-based and sustainable development approaches into the transnational feminist agenda. They argued that advocacy for women's rights should go beyond donor and NGO assistance to coalition building and to lobbying governments, corporations, and international banks. Through the tireless work of women's groups, transnational feminist advocacy pushed for "intersectional gendered perspectives" to "become central to human rights, environment, population, and sustainable development discourses in and around the United Nations," and they are responsible for "the emergence of a global gender equality regime" (Desai 2015: 125).

However, by the late 1990s, several factors begin to push back on transnational feminist organizing and its global gender equality regime. In 1991, the Soviet Union collapsed, ending the Cold War. After this, the U.S. gained its status as the singular global leader and even more influence in international institutions. Over the next few decades, representatives of the U.S. slowly shifted away from the collectivist interpretations of feminist empowerment that called for systemic change, which were popular with women's groups in the Soviet Union and the Global South. Aid programs addressing women's empowerment became narrower, often based on economic entrepreneurship or an individual's educational achievements (Radhakrishnan and Solari 2025).

Additionally, the above argument that gender equality should be integrated into numerous development sectors was used to justify gender mainstreaming. Gender mainstreaming attempts to integrate gender equality activities into development projects conducted by NGOs in all sectors, such as education, health, or agriculture. Mainstreaming has mixed results in its ability to fully address gender equality issues, which can often be sidelined for the sector that is an organization's focus. Mainstreaming also limited funding for organizations directly focused on women's issues and therefore feminist organizations around the world have been shrinking since 1995 (Goetz 2020; Okech and Musindarwezo 2019; Ransom and Bain 2011; Tripp 2006).

Finally, by the 1990s, we see the rise of a strong backlash movement. In 1994, at the UN International Conference on Population, the Vatican brought together conservative countries, allying specifically with Iran and Libya at this conference, to reject development programming that attempted to upgrade women's autonomy over reproductive decisions. What started as a small backlash coalition has now become a global right-wing movement made up of those opposed to gender freedoms and aiming to protect traditional social virtues. Conservative groups from nations with very different ethnic and religious backgrounds have come together due to a shared hatred of feminism and opposition to topics like reproductive and LGBTQ+ rights. This backlash has gotten more visible in the most recent decade, with political leaders like the U.S.'s Donald Trump, Russia's Vladimir Putin, and India's Narendra Modi pushing for the "re-masculinization" of their nations and regions (Radhakrishnan and Solari 2023).

The backlash movement made transnational feminist organizing more difficult. At the 2012 UN Commission on the Status of Women (UN Women), backlash groups blocked sexual education initiatives. During the writing of the UN's Sustainable Development Goals in 2015, the NGO, Group of Friends and Family, backed by conservative states and the Vatican, pushed back on activities geared towards changing men's roles in the household. Transnational feminist groups decided not to hold a fifth world conference on women for fear that these groups would hinder advancement on gender equality (Goetz 2020). In 2023, UN Women reported that progress towards Sustainable Development Goal Three, achieving gender equality by 2030, is off track due to institutional barriers, bias, unequal political representation, economic disparities, and a lack of legal protections for women (Robinson 2023).

Despite backlash, at least for now, gender equality and women's empowerment remain key areas of aid intervention. Transnational feminist groups continue to advocate in different forums such as the UN Human Rights Council and the Population Council (Goetz 2020). Aid projects promoting gender equality are implemented as part of assistance programs from global banks such as the International Monetary Fund (IMF) and the World Bank. Every OECD member country provides at least some funding aid for gender equality or women's empowerment (OECD 2022). In 2020, the OECD's official development committee reported that, of the total foreign aid provided by member countries, 45 percent either integrated women's empowerment or gender equality into its work through mainstreaming or was entirely dedicated to those topics (OECD 2020). To promote gender equality through aid, donors and INGOs intervene in numerous sectors, but support for maternal and reproductive health is one of the most prominent.

Gender, Development, and Health

Good health and well-being, in general, is the UN's third Sustainable Development Goal and a key sector for which foreign aid donors provide funding. The Global North has been intervening in the healthcare practices of nations in the Global South since colonization. In 1851, the International Sanitary Conventions began in France to regulate the spread of diseases so that epidemics did not impede global trade. The World Health Organization (WHO), with its organizational mission to promote health globally, was founded in 1948, shortly after World War II (White 2023). Nevertheless, it is in the second half of the twentieth century, in response to new disease threats like HIV, SARS, drug resistant TB, and, most recently, COVID-19, that we see global health funding grow tremendously. Donor funds for global health went from 5.8 billion in 1990 to 27.7 billion in 2011 (Packard 2016). In 2022, for OECD member nations, over 9 percent of the 56-billion-dollar development assistance budget went to upgrading healthcare in the Global South (OECD 2022). Due in large part to the feminist organizing described above, two key areas for global health funding are maternal health and family planning.

Transnational feminist advocacy groups contend that improvements to both maternal and reproductive healthcare are key to advancing the position of women globally (Davis 2007). They have good reason to do so as maternal and reproductive health programs can improve the lives of women, children, and families. Long-standing research shows that contraceptive access and its use improves the health of women and their children. Preventing unwanted pregnancies decreases maternal mortality and increases women's overall health. Contraceptive access also enables women to gain higher levels of education and pursue opportunities in the labor market. Finally, having fewer children allows families to better financially and emotionally support the ones they do have, and fewer unwanted pregnancies lead to less stunting and malnutrition in infants (Barot 2017).

The history of global aid for reproductive health and family planning is embedded in the history of transnational feminist interactions with the population control movement. After World War II, assistance for maternal health and family planning was intertwined with fears about unrestricted population growth in the Global South, worries about white fertility not keeping pace, and the dominant eugenics model of the time. The success of global and national efforts to curb infectious diseases meant fewer people were dying, but nothing had been done to limit population growth. To address this, the first World Population Council meeting was held in 1954 (Packard 2016).

Early population interventions faced strong pushback from Catholic countries and constituencies. This meant that in the 1950s most bilateral aid donors were hesitant to intervene in the area. Consequently, private foundations like Planned Parenthood and the World Population Council played a leading role in the first efforts to address the global population crisis and provide family planning methods to women in the Global South. By the 1960s, USAID and several European donors started channeling funding to these private foundations and NGOs working in population control. Working through nongovernmental actors in this sector enabled donor nations to lessen the appearance of intervention into the population growth of other countries and avoid backlash from their own Catholic populations (Packard 2016).

By the early 1970s, feminist groups begin to take issue with the population control model, which had illustrated limited effectiveness and a lack of care for women's rights (Packard 2016). Transnational feminist advocacy on the topic of family planning was consolidated through numerous international conferences and transnational networks, as well as interactions with the population control organizations, gaining massive traction by the 1980s (Petchesky 2003). Several events help transnational women's groups gain cross-border coalitions on the topic of women's health. In 1970 the first copy of *Our Bodies, Ourselves* challenged medical dogma about women's health and taught women about their bodies. It sold more than four million copies and was translated into multiple languages through the 1980s and 1990s (Davis 2007). Additionally, in the 1970s, due to feminist organizing, contraceptive pills and abortion were being legalized across Europe and in the U.S. At this time, Western feminists advocated for the right to family planning and female choice in the decision to bear children globally. By 1977, the first International Women's Health meeting was held in Rome to mobilize groups around the world to address women's health issues (Turshen 2020).

However, following the earlier pattern of North-South tensions, by the International Women's Health meeting in Geneva in 1981, women's groups from the Global South came in with a strong critique of Western women's advocacy. They were critical of population control programming and Western women's emphasis on the freedom of choice not to bear children. They took issue with the fact that women's groups in the Global North ignored how reproductive health agendas can constrain marginalized people's birthing choices (Littlejohn 2021; Suh 2021). For women in the Global South, population control programs, with their eugenics legacies, were frequently stopping them from having children, even when they wanted to do so. Women's groups brought the right to motherhood into the conversation about global women's health advocacy (Bracke 2023).

This argument for the right to motherhood was spurred on by high maternal mortality rates in the Global South. Transnational feminist organizations for women's health brought these rates to the attention of global aid donors. In 1987, the UN, the World Health Organization, and the World Bank sponsored the Safe Motherhood Conference in Nairobi. The conference increased global focus on maternal health, drawing attention to the half million maternal deaths that occur each year and the fact that birthing people in the Global South run 50–100 times the risk of dying in childbirth compared to those in the Global North (Starrs 2006). By 2010, at the thirty-sixth G8 summit, member nations collectively committed to spend 5 billion U.S. dollars in five years to address maternal and infant mortality through the Muskoka Initiative on Maternal, Newborn, and Child Health. Member nations committed more funding to a second Muskoka Initiative in 2014 (Banchani and Swiss 2019).

Women's health activists also mobilized to put health on the agenda at the UN's women's conferences and population conferences. Due to this advocacy, the conclusions of the 1985 UN Women's Conference in Nairobi included a statement on reproductive health and rights as essential preconditions for the improvement of women's social status. It also called on governments to implement a series of laws and policies enabling medical infrastructure and training for healthcare workers to better address women's health needs (Bracke 2023). The 1995 Beijing Women's Conference included women's health as a key area of concern along with strategic actions to address gender disparities (UN 2020).

Throughout the 1990s, transnational feminist groups also succeed in getting prominent foundations that provided funding for population control to examine the gendered impact of their work (Petchesky 2003). The 1994 UN International Conference on Population and Development in Cairo is considered a watershed moment for transnational women's health organizing (Garita 2015). At this time, transnational activists succeeded in shifting the global rhetoric around population control from a demographic need for economic development to a gender lens that recognizes reproductive health as an essential path for women's empowerment (Bracke 2023; Petchesky 2003).

However, as we saw above, sexual and reproductive health are key topics in which the global antigender backlash movement has intervened, stymieing progress towards women's health goals. On the international scene, women's groups faced pushback from conservative groups at many conferences. In 1985, President Reagan first implemented the Mexico City Policy, which banned INGOs that provided abortion counseling from receiving USAID funding (Petroni and Skuster 2008). Due to the politicized nature of abortion in the U.S., the Mexico City Policy has been subsequently removed and then reinstated with successive changes in presidential administrations.

Despite setbacks, transnational women's health groups continued to push forward. During the 2011 UN General Assembly in Mexico City, feminist, human rights, and youth organizations pushed for the "Our Rights, Our Lives" call to action. This call included the demand for universal health access, including reproductive care, the adoption of sexual rights as human rights, and programs that empower youth and adolescents to better understand their sexual health (Garita 2015).

Today, all OECD members provide funding to maternal health. Maternal and newborn health are particularly popular aid interventions across the political spectrum. Before its recent shutdown, USAID's website declared in bold letters "Ending preventable maternal and child deaths is within reach," and JICA's website states that maternal and child health programming "protects precious lives." Many OECD countries also frequently provide maternal health programs in an integrated fashion with family planning activities. For instance, in 2022, the U.S. global health budget was almost 13 billion dollars. Of that, about 1.5 billion went to maternal and child health and another 600 million went to family planning activities (KFF 2023).

Throughout the latter half of the twentieth century, maternal mortality dropped around the world. However, in 2020, an estimated 830 women still died due to pregnancy-related causes globally each day (Turshen 2020). In response, women's health groups from the Global South have tried to push for a discussion about how the larger global economic system shapes women's health outcomes. Countries that have enacted structural adjustment policies have seen detrimental impacts to maternal and child health. Issues like lack of access to affordable healthcare, nutrition, stable incomes, and clean water radically shape women's health outcomes (Kentikelenis and Stubbs 2023; Petchesky 2003; Turshen 2020). Women's groups have pushed back against short-term results-oriented donor projects, donor agendas that ignore a recipient nation's healthcare strategy, and a focus on reproductive healthcare solely as a method for women's integration into the labor market (Mallik et al. 2023; Plummer, Smith, and Hughes 2018). Such critiques lead us to a discussion of the changing nature of aid for gender equality and women's health in the international development sector today.

NGOs in Crisis?

International and local NGOs have been engaging in aid activities around gender, healthcare, and other social inequalities since the NGO boom of the 1990s. NGO advocacy has increased donor and government healthcare spending with favorable effects on health outcomes in many recipient nations. The presence of NGOs is also associated with improved acceptance of

LGBTQ+ people and improvement of women's economic position in many cases. Studies in several nations have illustrated that citizens in contact with NGOs are more likely to be politically engaged. Finally, NGO advocacy has also played a key role in the emergence of new state institutions, like women's ministries or maternal child health agencies (Brass 2021; Schmitz and Mitchell 2022).

In contrast, NGOs struggle to increase women's leadership roles in politics. The presence of NGOs and activities geared towards improving gender equality can also create domestic backlash movements (Pike 2019). Additionally, NGO service provision can crowd out government services, decreasing citizen use of public services (Schmitz and Mitchell 2022). Finally, many criticize NGO activities for enacting the individualist and economically centered version of empowerment described above, limiting collective mobilization or structural change (Bernal and Grewal 2014).

Why such mixed results? In part, it is due to the variety of roles NGOs enact in undertaking both advocacy and service provision. As we saw above, in their advocacy role, NGOs are often the organizational form which local women's groups enact to sustain themselves, gaining access to donor funding and transnational networks. NGOs can provide the space for communities to contest, not just global agendas, but also local cultural norms, unjust policies, and/or institutions that contribute to social inequalities (Davis 2007; Noonan 2002; Thayer 2010). For instance, foreign aid interventions that worked to raise awareness about and prevent HIV in India unintentionally opened an institutionalized space for sexual minority groups to advocate for their rights (Vijayakumar 2021).

But many NGOs focus on service provision or education, not advocacy or mobilization. For example, in Senegal, aid activities aiming to decrease maternal mortality unintentionally resulted in the number of unsafe abortions being obscured (Suh 2021). Aid activities to advance gender equality and healthcare simply have varying impacts depending on the nature of the activities and recipient contexts. Whether the outcomes of aid interventions are liberatory for women is deeply influenced by a recipient nation's existing institutions, economic organization, and cultural context (Klausen 2015; Mojola 2014; Noonan 2002; Tavory and Swidler 2009).

The findings from Senegal also bring up a further problem that NGOs face—in some case donor demands can constrain the capacity of NGO workers to adapt programs to local needs (Dionne 2018; Swidler and Watkins 2017; Suh 2021). NGO connections to foreign donors can make it difficult for them to both meet the demands of recipient populations and maintain donor interests (Schmitz and Mitchell 2022; Spires 2012; Swidler and Watkins 2017). In response, we increasingly see calls for NGOs and donors to "decolonize" and center the needs of people in the Global South (Turshen 2020). Due to these mixed results, the effectiveness of NGOs is now in question, and some donors are moving away from these organizations. However, to fully understand the changes the NGO sector is facing, we must look at the larger transformations taking place in the foreign aid system.

Foreign Aid in the Context of Global Transformations

Foreign aid organizations are key players in the creation and dispersal of international development models. Development models "are forged by development experts working in the Ivory Tower and multilateral organizations, but also by states, which can play a major role in selecting, interpreting, and packaging development facts. Wealthy, powerful states may deliberately export particular development models, based on particular understandings of past events, through both multilateral institutions and bilateral foreign-aid programs" (Taniguchi and Babb 2009: 278). After the Cold War, we saw this exportation with the convergence of foreign aid around a U.S.-led, neoliberal development model.

Yet, as discussed in the introduction, the 2008 financial crisis and disillusionment with the social consequences of structural adjustment have led to declining confidence in the neoliberal economic development model promoted by the U.S. and the U.K. (Woods 2008). Increasing economic inequality and concerns about global economic transformations in the West have contributed to the rising attractiveness of populist leaders on the far right, who frequently advocate for isolationism, crackdowns on immigration, and nationalism (Radhakrishnan and Solari 2023; Silver 2022). Populist political leaders advocate for Western nations to reduce global engagement and foreign aid. For instance, before her conviction, French far-right populist leader Marine Le Pen argued that economic globalization and Islamic fundamentalism were the enemies of France (Ivaldi 2024). The U.S. also reelected President Trump in 2024. Trump's "America First" rhetoric is strongly antiglobalization, and one of his early executive orders in January 2025 was to shut down USAID, which will be discussed in the conclusion of this book. These isolationist, antiglobal strategies are contributing to a decline in the long-held soft power of the U.S. and Europe in the international development sector (Regilme 2023).

Meanwhile, we are seeing emerging donors like China, India, and Brazil challenging the dominant foreign aid model, offering different financing and assistance models, and providing alternative paths for development (Wyrod 2019). In 2011, the OECD Forum on Aid Effectiveness was held in Busan, South Korea. There, emerging donors pushed for a development agenda focused on economic and infrastructure development as well as "South-South" partnerships (Mawdsley, Savage, and Kim 2014). The emergence of "new" or non-OECD member donors is changing the relationships between donors, NGOs, recipient states, and beneficiaries (Roth 2015). As emerging donors offer alternative funding models to recipient nations, they have introduced competitive pressures into the traditional OECD aid system. In recent decades recipient nations have been calling for more government ownership over aid programs, and many see emerging donors, who are less likely to impose conditions on aid, as a possible solution (Woods 2008).

Alongside these donor transformations—and despite important national variation and competition between donors from East Asia—China, Japan, and South Korea have been engaging in regionalized rhetoric about an Asian development model since the early 2000s (Kondoh et al. 2010; Stallings and Kim 2017). Due to its rising economic dominance, China is a powerful emerging donor and a key player in promoting a new model of development. China has massively expanded its aid program in the Global South in recent decades. In 2023, it was assisting 140 nations and providing approximately 350 billion U.S. dollars in aid. In contrast to the traditional OECD model, less than 25 percent of Chinese aid has a grant component, with most Chinese aid coming in the form of loans and infrastructure development as well as commercial and trade deals (Regilme 2003). Xi Jinping, the president of China, has named China "the leader of the Global South" and plans to use Chinese aid to make this a reality (Kilby 2017; Regilme 2023).

Together with its aid, China promotes the alternative of adopting Asian Confucian values, in contrast to the Western liberal ones that have been dispersed like individualism, gender equality, and competitiveness (Kilby 2017; Regilme 2023). Consequently, China is "providing a rival vision of development and good governance in aid recipient countries in the Global

South" (Regilme 2023: 47). However, Global South recipient responses to Chinese aid are decidedly mixed (Blair, Marty, and Roessler 2022).

Japan, as the first East Asian nation to industrialize, is an OECD member and not considered an emerging donor. Nevertheless, it also plays a key role in the promotion of an alternative "Asian" development model. Foreign aid from Japan began in the late 1950s. Japan paid reparations to four countries in Southeast Asia—Myanmar, the Philippines, Indonesia, and Vietnam. Soon after, Japan began to offer loans, small grants, and technical assistance to numerous Southeast Asian nations (JICA 2013; Er 2013). Aid to Southeast Asia helped Japan to rehabilitate its image in the region and promote Japanese foreign investment (Higuchi 2013). Additionally, South Korea was originally considered a prominent emerging donor (Woods 2008). It set up its bilateral agency in 1991 and by 1996 decided to join the OECD as a global development partner (Egan and Persaud 2021).

As OECD members, Japan and South Korea are subject to following Official Development Committee standards. Yet Japan and South Korea also draw on regional frameworks similar to that of China (Kilby 2017; Mawdsley, Savage, and Kim 2014). Japan was the first East Asian nation to articulate an "East Asian" development model to challenge the Washington Consensus in the 1980s (Taniguchi and Babb 2009). In the Japanese development sector today, practitioners promote Japan's prominence as East Asia's first donor, contending that aid donors in South Korea and China should follow Japan's lead. South Korean leaders also speak out about the importance of Asian cooperation in the global order, and most assistance from the Korean International Cooperation Agency (KOICA), South Korea's bilateral agency, goes to Asian nations (SEEK Development 2023).

In summary, there has been a rise in far-right populist leaders in the U.S. and Europe that want to shift the purpose of aid from helping the neediest around the world to serving more of their own economic and political ends. Alongside this, there is an Asian development model that provides grant aid less frequently and instead promotes economic and infrastructure development (Regilme 2023; Stallings and Kim 2017). These circumstances are decreasing the amount of funding NGOs receive. South Korea, China, and Japan engage with NGOs in a more limited fashion than traditional Western donors. China, well known for its suppression of or governmentalization of NGOs in its own country, does not fund NGOs in its foreign aid at all (Spires 2012). Japan provides between 1 and 3 percent of its total ODA (official development assistance) budget only to Japan-based INGOs, which was a total of 15.7 billion U.S. dollars in funding in 2021 (OECD 2021). This contrasts with Western donors, which fund INGOs based all over the world. When I inquire about the choice to fund only Japanese INGOs in Tokyo, JICA interviewees explain that it is important that peoples in recipient nations "see the face of Japan."

KOICA does have a Civil Society Cooperation budget that provides funding to NGOs. However, in 2019, only approximately 22,000 US dollars went to civil society funding out of KOICA's ODA budget of 2.61 billion US dollars (KOICA 2020; SEEK Development 2023). Additionally, in my own fieldwork I discovered that, in 2016, KOICA's Cambodia office provided funding to local NGOs in Phnom Penh through its Civil Society Cooperation program. However, by 2017, KOICA interviewees in Phnom Penh said their organization had changed direction and decided to only provide funding to Korean INGOs, following the lead of JICA. Thus, KOICA's cooperation with NGOs is still in flux and is itself influenced by the regionalization of aid donors.

Finally, isolationism and regionalization are also changing the nature of aid norms for health and gender. In general, there is rising regionalization and interregional referencing taking place in development organizations that work in the health sector (Lange 2020; Onzivu 2012). The COVID-19 pandemic illustrated the limits of the World Health Organization's power to stop the global spread of disease. In response, many governments turned towards regional organizations to protect their citizens. For instance, Australia and Japan funded Asia-Pacific health initiatives to try to curb the spread of COVID-19. Consequently, many speculate we are moving away from global governance towards a polycentric model of global health governance. This trend was only spurred on by President Trump's recent decision to leave the WHO (Lange 2020).

Additionally, as we saw above, due to transnational feminist advocacy, gender equality has been a goal of traditional foreign aid donors. Gendered beliefs—including the positions of men and women in the economy, family, and politics—are all battlefields on which national leaders, donors, and development practitioners contest what it means to advance society and women's place within it (Lynch 2007). We can see this in my coworker Lakena's negotiation with distinctive donor beliefs about the best way to advance women.

Yet, the capture of state power by far-right conservative groups has furthered backlash against gender equality (Petchesky 2003; Radhakrishnan

and Solari 2023). Many East Asian donors also have distinctive aid practices when it comes to gender equality when compared to the traditionally
dominant donors from the U.S. and Europe. Japan's aid has often skirted
around the OECD demand to enhance gender equality and/or civil society,
balancing surface-level commitment to placate traditional donors alongside a desire to invest in "nonpolitical" gender projects like maternal health
(Ichihara 2013).

Other donors, like China, efface the topic of gender all together. For
instance, while World Bank projects frequently increase local support for
gender equality, studies show Chinese aid in the same areas does not have
the same effect (Zhang and Huang 2023). Yet one cannot implement aid
projects addressing topics like maternal health without intervening in wom-
en's roles in work and family. Consequently, women's health programs are
an important site where the effects of foreign aid regionalization need to be
examined.

The above studies of regionalization and foreign aid have largely been
conducted in international meetings or at the donor level, documenting
new models of development (Kilby 2017; Lange 2020; Mawdsley, Savage,
and Kim 2014). But, as the research on NGOs and localization in recipient
contexts has illustrated, development models are not constructed only by
powerful actors from wealthier nations. Practitioners in recipient nations
articulate donor demands into aid practices and modify donor interpretations of international development. Subsequent chapters present a study of
the regionalization of foreign aid from below.

From Strategic Alliances to Unruly Recipients
Women's Health and INGO-State Partnerships

A USAID-funded INGO is hosting a women's health conference in Phnom Penh. In attendance are at least two hundred people—donor representatives, NGO staffers, government officials, and public and private health clinic workers. A high-ranking Ministry of Health official kicks off the event with a lengthy speech. She exclaims that it is time for the Cambodian government to "be strong" and "take the lead" in maternal and child health. She asks the audience, "Do we want donors to decide what is best for our children? Our mothers? Our families?" The air in the room gets tense as she chides the public health officials in attendance for "sitting back" and "taking orders from international donors." She explains that while foreign donors helped Cambodia immensely after the Khmer Rouge, the Ministry of Health has grown in its capacity, and no longer needs to be "led around" by donor agendas. As her speech draws to a close, she calls for Cambodia to take the lead in its national health implementation and show itself to be a strong Asian nation.

Since the 1990s, foreign donors have contributed ample resources and technical knowledge to the Cambodian public health sector and to other government agencies. However, currently, many Cambodian officials, like the minister above, believe it is time for Cambodians to wrest control of the government back from foreign aid donors. As we see in the minister's speech, this involves control over decisions about the way that the state should intervene in gender and family relations. State interventions have the power to restructure the dynamics of gender and family in a country.

This means topics like motherhood or women's workforce participation frequently become central to debates about what would advance a society (Connell 1990; Puri 2003). For instance, in the U.S., political debates about legal access to abortion engage different conceptions of the role women should play as mothers and workers in modern American society (Luker 1985). Similarly, this chapter illustrates how competing development imaginaries are used to articulate the role that the state should play in women's health.

This chapter investigates the partnerships between Cambodian public health agencies and the two INGOs in this study, Japan Services Asia (JSA) and U.S. Family Aid (USFA). Within each INGO's donor gender regime are different understandings of the role developing states and the market should play in distributing health services to women. Japan Services Asia centers the government as the provider of maternal health services. In contrast, U.S. Family Aid tends to see the market and nonprofit sector as the primary distributors of women's health services, with the state coordinating nonstate actors. In response to these two models, Cambodian development practitioners and public health officials mobilize the development imaginaries to craft distinctive partnerships. However, before discussing these two cases in depth, we need to examine why both JSA and USFA decide to work in partnership with the Cambodian state in the first place.

Why Partner with the Cambodian State?

While their partnerships may be different, both INGOs see cooperation with the Cambodian state as a road to creating a sustainable impact. Yet, the fact that both INGOs in this study cooperate with the Cambodian state may be surprising at first, given the conventional assumptions about the role NGOs play in development. States are a key site where bilateral and multilateral donors have intervened, and struggles take place over foreign and domestic interests (Ferguson 2021). However, traditionally, international and local NGOs are assumed to be "nongovernmental," as their name suggests, or civil society actors. Historically, NGOs have frequently been understood as a space for citizens to advocate for their interests or provide for underserved populations. On its website, the United Nations defines NGOs as part of the "third sector," separate from both states and private actors.[1] This definition is not unfounded as many NGOs do enact a nonstate role, either by providing services without state cooperation or by mobilizing grassroots groups to advocate to states, corporations, or international organizations for change (Ferree and Tripp 2006).

Nevertheless, in the past twenty years, development cooperation between NGOs and states has grown more frequent (Banks, Hulme, and Edwards 2015; Brass 2016). This is particularly true for NGO projects that aim to upgrade healthcare (Hushie 2016). Specifically, this push for cooperation between NGOs, states, and donors became stronger after the United Nations Conference on Sustainable Development in Rio de Janeiro in 2012. The Rio conference initiated a working group to create a new set of development goals (updating the Millennium Development Goals). Outspoken leaders from several nations in the Global South advocated for changes that would address previous inequalities in the implementation of the UN's Millennium Development Goals (Caballero 2019).

Challenging previous assumptions that development goals were only applicable in developing countries, leaders from the Global South contended that the new goals needed to be truly global and pursued in all countries. This argument came alongside strong encouragement for developed nations to cooperate with developing countries as equal partners when providing aid. After much debate, the Sustainable Development Goals (SDGs) were formally adopted by the UN in 2015. The promotion of equal partnership is particularly prominent in the third SDG, "good health and well-being," which includes the target to strengthen the capacity of developing states. This goal advocates the need for bringing governments back in to achieve the goal of making healthcare affordable for all (Ranabhat et al. 2023).

After the adoption of the SDGs, INGOs increasingly faced pressure from the United Nations and donor organizations to partner with developing nations. This push for equal partnership was only strengthened by emerging donors like China and India. Emerging donors often claim to engage in South-South partnerships with recipient states to determine their aid agendas, which are more equitable than partnerships with traditional donors (Mawdsley, Savage, and Kim 2014). While Japanese NGOs have historically cooperated closely with recipient states, this push meant many U.S.-based INGOs needed to stop bypassing the state to work with private health actors or provide services solely through NGOs. Consequently, we can no longer assume that NGOs are always distinctly civic actors isolated from the state or market. This chapter interrogates how distinctive

NGO-state partnerships are created through interactions between donors, practitioners, and state actors (Brass 2016; Lichterman and Eliasoph 2014; Viterna, Clough, and Clarke 2015).

To understand each INGO's partnership, it is also important to remember that states are not singular entities. Different government agencies can pursue varying agendas and exhibit diverse levels of administrative capacity (Ferguson 2021; Li 2005; McDonnell 2020; Morgan and Orloff 2017). In Cambodia, the public health system is multitiered. First, the Ministry of Health is the leading force in planning, developing, and overseeing the national health system. Then, the country is broken up into twenty-four provinces, so the Ministry of Health oversees the provincial health department and provincial hospital in each of the nation's provinces. Next, each provincial health department oversees the district health departments and district referral hospitals (WHO 2016).

Districts are then broken into communes. District health departments oversee health centers and health posts in their communes. There are an estimated 1,105 health centers in the country.[2] Most health centers are equipped to provide primary care, maternal and child health services, and the prevention of communicable diseases. Finally, at the village level, ideally, health centers oversee and provide a small allowance to village health volunteers who act as health educators at the village level. Figure 2 illustrates the Cambodian public health system.

The Cambodian health system also includes private options for care. There are approximately 2,000 private health clinics in Cambodia. All pri-

FIGURE 2. The Cambodian Health System.

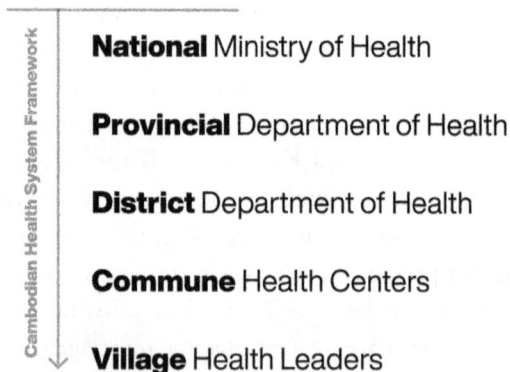

Cambodian Health System Framework

National Ministry of Health

Provincial Department of Health

District Department of Health

Commune Health Centers

Village Health Leaders

vate health clinics and drugstores are legally required to register with the Ministry of Health. However, in 2010, only about half were registered and even private health clinics that are registered remain largely unregulated by the government (Hwang, Seap, and Kim 2016; WHO 2016). Additionally, many doctors that work in the public sector also run or work for private clinics (Khim et al. 2020).

JSA and USFA both enter partnerships with the Cambodian state. However, each INGO selects a different state agency as its partner and chooses distinctive activities to implement. Below, I detail (1) each INGO's state partnership model, (2) the state organization it selects as a partner, (3) each INGO's partnership activities, and, finally, (4) how partnerships are reinforced or resisted by Cambodian practitioners and state officials.

Japan Services Asia: The State-as-Distributor Model

It is a cool morning in the small town of Sesan, in the northern province of Steung Treng, where the Japanese INGO, Japan Services Asia (JSA), has its provincial office. I sit in the open-air, two-room office as fans blow around papers and staff assemble around a large table. Stray chickens, cats, and dogs wander in and out of the office. JSA's Japanese director, Junko, and her Japanese intern, Hanako, sit in conversation with the organization's Cambodian, male managerial staff, Boran, Samnang, Chhy, and Sovann. They discuss their strategy for building a successful government partnership. They are working on identifying and befriending another official in the Steung Treng provincial health department, their main state partner agency, who has enough influence to ensure staff from the provincial health department attend JSA's workshops.

Junko and Boran list off different doctors in the provincial health department by name. Boran poses to the group, "What about Dr. Mao?" Junko responds she is not sure he has a sufficient level of influence for a government liaison. When Boran next suggests Dr. In, Samnang expresses skepticism about Dr. In's level of commitment to implementing public health policies. Hearing this, Junko becomes defiant: "In response to disinterest, we must make them move just as we did in Kampong Speu [their previous project site]. We can offer support for what they need—conferences, per diems, meetings, and slowly, slowly we will build the right connections." She passionately exclaims that they must convince public health officials to follow the Ministry of Health's policy, attend JSA trainings, and implement health services for mothers and newborns. "It is their job to implement the MOH [Ministry of Health] policy! Don't they know it is their job?"

Junko and her program managers focus considerable energy on making the right connections in the government. This is because Japan's gender regime centers the government as the provider of maternal health services or what I call the *state-as-distributor* model. If you will recall from the introduction, a gender regime is the way in which donor projects are embedded within and diffuse their own nation's dominant gendered beliefs through distinctive interventions into Cambodia's state, civil society, and private sector (Connell 1990). The push for the state as distributor of women's health services is evident in the development sector in Tokyo. With strong state leadership, Japan developed rapidly and made massive improvements to its public healthcare and education system in the 1950s and 1960s. Japan uses foreign aid to promote its own rapid development as an example for nations in the Global South to follow.

Japanese donors fund projects that support the creation of a developmental state in numerous recipient nations (Arase 2005; Tonami 2018). Practitioners in Tokyo describe the state as the primary agent of development. One interviewee says, "the Japanese government . . . provide[s] needed services to Japanese people, like medical services, education, all of it. So, in the past, we don't need to think about those. I think the people in the developing countries deserve to have those services too."

In terms of women's health, JICA interviewees in Tokyo contend aid-receiving countries can particularly learn from Japan's own successful maternal and child public health system. Japan has one of the most highly developed public maternal health systems in the world alongside some of the lowest maternal mortality rates. Japanese aid focuses on exporting key factors in Japan's success such as "women-only professions" (training courses for nurses and midwives), training public health workers, the development of a Maternal and Child Health Handbook, and increasing the number and quality of public birthing centers (JICA 2005: 73).

For example, during my time in Tokyo, I was invited to observe a JICA-funded training on maternal health. I sat in the back of the large training room with multiple JICA officials. In front of us sat eight public health officials from Niger, Sierra Leone, Uganda, and Namibia. Five are male and three are female. The JICA official leading their trip to Japan explains to me the participants are all trained as midwives or doctors. Each participant was nominated by their government to attend the training in Japan. After workshops in Tokyo, the group will be traveling to different prefectures around Japan to observe maternal healthcare implementation.

For the first half of the workshop, the Japanese trainer provides officials with information about post- and prenatal care, delivery standards, maternal nutrition, and newborn nutrition. Then, the trainer begins a discussion about how trainees can ensure the improvement of government maternal and child health policies. First, she asks, "What did Japan do?" pulling up a PowerPoint where the first slide is titled "Japanese experience from the top and bottom." She explains Japan's maternal child health history, including the training of public nurses, the Maternal and Child Health Handbook, and government healthcare infrastructure. To illustrate Japan's rapid development, she shows black-and-white photos of postwar Japan in comparison to bright cityscape photos of today's Tokyo.

Trainees discuss how Japan's policies can or cannot be used in their countries. They express concern their governments "will not move without payment" or might lack the resources to implement Japan-style maternal child healthcare. The trainer largely glosses over these concerns, urging trainees to "be creative and persistent." Trainees are tasked with "planning an effective advocacy strategy." They do so by discussing how to build relationships with decision-makers in government, how to frame their message around the "universal good" of improving the health of mothers and young children, and the need to convince "their friends" in the national government. In this training, we can see clearly that, in Tokyo, women's health needs are addressed through the strong promotion of the Japanese maternal health experience.

Consequently, JSA's main goal in its state partnership is to upgrade the capacity of the Cambodian state to provide maternal health services. While the content of maternal health activities will be discussed more directly in chapter 3, this chapter focuses on the INGO-state partnership created by JSA practitioners and Cambodian state officials under this model. Nevertheless, using the state-as-distributor model means JSA's state partnership comes with two gendered assumptions about who can access and who provides care. First, it asserts that all mothers should have access to affordable, quality public healthcare for pregnancy and childbirth. But it ignores inequities that may arise from a largely male-dominated public health sector in Cambodia.[3]

PARTNER AGENCY SELECTION

Because it uses a distributor model, when constructing its project activities, JSA selects the provincial and district health departments in Steung Treng as its partner agencies. Steung Treng is a remote, rural province about five to six hours north of Cambodia's capital city, Phnom Penh. JSA maintains a provincial office in a small district town, Scsan, where state presence is quite limited. The town is about an hour away from the provincial capital of Steung Treng. Power outages are frequent and only some of the wooden houses in town have running water. Steung Treng is a province with some of the worst indicators for maternal health, nutrition for expectant mothers and children under two, and poverty. The clear need in the province for improved public health services makes it appealing to JSA's donors. JSA's director, Junko, explains that maintaining an office in this area (alongside their Phnom Penh office) allows her staff to be on the ground in a province where the Provincial Health Department might be willing to implement health services but lacks capacity to do so at this time.

Explaining how JSA selected this site for its provincial office, Junko points to the Cambodian Ministry of Health's "Health Strategic Plan," which JICA played an important role in writing. According to the plan, the provincial and district levels are considered the main implementers of the ministry's policies, not unlike Japan's prefectures, which are the main implementers in Japan's healthcare system. Before the project began, Junko and Boran traveled to Steung Treng to build relationships with the provincial health department officials, who then recommended specific districts where JSA might focus its efforts. At JSA, state partnership comes with the assumptions that social ties are key to project success.

Most INGOs are not willing to open offices in remote provincial locations, as middle-class NGO staff prefer to live in Phnom Penh, Siem Reap (Cambodia's second-largest city), or, at the very least, provincial capital cities. Typically, INGOs from the U.S., Europe, and Australia fund local NGOs to implement programming in rural areas. However, Japanese practitioners in Tokyo and Cambodia interpret the call for development organizations to do "grassroots" activities as requiring close cooperation with local-level government officials.

When giving a new staff orientation, Boran puts up a PowerPoint. After detailing JSA's mission and history, he describes the current project. He pulls up a slide with a bullet point stating, "JSA's devotion to working on the grassroots level," next to a model of the different decentralized levels of the Cambodian government. Initially, I am confused by this; as an American, the term "grassroots" suggests civil society or community advocacy to me. Yet, without missing a beat, Boran explains that to work on the grassroots level means cooperation with multiple subnational government partners. Grassroots partners are considered nonnational officials, from the provincial, district, and commune levels.

In Tokyo, I discover that this understanding of the term "grassroots" is widespread. Japanese INGO staff often tell me that their organization works at the grassroots level and then proceed to describe their partnerships with local-level government officials. An INGO program manager states, "Yes, we work at the grassroots level, with the district officials, commune leaders, and government village volunteers." Moreover, a bilateral agency interviewee informs me that JICA's INGO partnership program is called the *kusanone* (the Japanese word for grassroots) program, in which INGOs are encouraged to engage in "grassroots technical cooperation with local government staff and stakeholders." Consequently, although JSA does maintain a small office in Phnom Penh, JSA selects a provincial government agency to be its main partner, and staff spend most of their time in Steung Treng to be near the relevant provincial and district officials.

Kaori, a JSA headquarters staff member visiting from Tokyo, reports that the long-term vision of JSA is that after successful implementation of maternal health services in Steung Treng, JSA will support provincial officials in documenting their improved maternal and child health outcomes. Then, alongside government partners, JSA staff will promote Steung Treng as a successful model for improving the public health system's capacity to distribute services at the national level so it can be expanded into more provinces.

PARTNERSHIP ACTIVITIES

JSA's program documents expressly state that JSA will improve the health of mothers and children in Steung Treng by increasing state capacity to monitor the nutrition and health of mothers and children. In part, accomplishing this goal takes the form of the "training of trainers" model. This means training higher-level government staff to provide health education training to subnational officials in the ranks below them. This training model, in which, for instance, a doctor might train nurses, and then nurses would train community volunteers, is not new in development practice. However, the way JSA deploys this model displays its centralized emphasis on state partnership.[4]

For the training of the trainers workshops, staff work closely with the head of the provincial maternal child health department, Dr. Kim. For the first workshop, we meet with Dr. Kim to plan how he will enhance the capacity of district-level state staff. The next day, provincial staff help train three district health officials from JSA's partner districts. JSA managers and Dr. Kim support district staff in preparing posters and presentations on maternal and child health information.

The next week, at JSA's office, Dr. Kim and the three district officials make these presentations at a workshop provided for health center mid-wives, nurses, and doctors from health centers in different communes in JSA's target areas. After this training, JSA then supports a fourth level of trainings, in which health center workers train village health volunteers on these topics in their own communes. For the fifth and final level of trainings, village health volunteers and health center workers implement community health trainings for mothers and pregnant women in villages. Here, JSA staff monitor that these trainings take place, run smoothly, and assist public health clinic staff with data collection on the number of pregnant women and young children in the villages.

During a village health training, as JSA program assistants help health center staff cajole babies onto scales to monitor their weight, Samnang and a health center worker instruct a village health volunteer who is about to give a breastfeeding and nutrition training. She asks, "six months only breastfeeding, is that correct?" Samnang answers affirmatively, briefly re-viewing the information with her before she begins her short presentation. Catching Samnang after the event, I inquire, why does he not give the training himself as most other NGOs do? He explains, this is a government activity—they need to do it—and he goes on to ask me rhetorically, if he did it for them, who will do it when JSA is gone? JSA helps the government to do its job.

In addition to trainings, JSA spends substantial time attending govern-ment meetings. While many INGOs have staff attend government meet-ings, they are typically strategic about which ones they attend. In contrast, JSA staff attend government meetings about two to five times per week. Sovann tells me about a commune planning meeting, where he briefed commune leaders about their budgets and how to access the funds available to them at the national bank. He reports the commune treasurers are not always well versed in banking matters, so he helps them understand how to access the funds. Then he gently informs them about JSA's data on maternal and child health to promote allocation of the commune budget towards community health programs. However, he "doesn't push this too hard," as it is also his job to get to know them and listen to their ideas. Sovann tells me, "if we give them too many ideas, next time, they might just listen to me and not have ideas of their own."

JSA's staff maintains an elaborate knowledge of state policies, takes a backseat role in implementation, and gently promotes maternal health policy implementation at government meetings. These activities illustrate the state-as-distributor model, assuming that in an ideal future, the public health system will be the main distributor of maternal health services. Next, I examine more closely how Cambodian practitioners and state officials use the development imaginary to reinforce and co-opt the state-as-distributor model at JSA.

Japan Services Asia and Development Imaginaries: Following the Path of Asia

INGO partnerships often come with the backing of powerful bilateral and multilateral agencies, and many nations in the Global South remain dependent on donors and INGOs to fill in gaps in social service provision. Nevertheless, while state officials in recipient nations may "bargain in the shadow of power," they still play an active role in strategically negotiating partnerships with international actors (Chorev 2020: 3). States in the Global South can constrain INGOs and donors by making laws restricting INGO activities, creating an unreceptive environment for partnership (Bromley, Schofer, and Longhofer 2019). In contrast, recipient states can cultivate partnerships by funding NGOs directly, seeking out partnerships in social service provision, or participating in NGO technical skills building workshops (Brass 2016; Kudva 2005). As we will see, state actors in the Global South actively negotiate and modify partnerships in their interactions with development practitioners.

REINFORCING AND RESONANCE

At the end of my observation at JSA, the staff held a party for me. After work hours, staff members cook *somlar kako*[5] (a Cambodian vegetable soup) on gas cooktops, barbeque meat, pick up beverages and ice from the local market, and set up tables and decorations in the dirt yard outside of the JSA office. We spend the evening drinking, eating, and singing together.

In attendance at this event were not just JSA staff members but also two district health doctors, a district governor, and the provincial health official, Dr. Kim. JSA's program managers and the provincial and district officials tell stories, sing, and laugh as they try to convince me to taste homemade herbal liquor. Program assistants help with food preparation, refill glasses, and sit together away from the men at the table. As foreigners, Junko and I are the only women who have a seat at the table.

Junko explains that JSA hires only male managers because doing so better enables her INGO to build connections with Cambodian public health officials, who are largely men. JSA managers then reinforce the state's distributor model alongside Cambodian state officials for three reasons. First, due to long tenure at JSA and a deep commitment to organizational goals, program managers themselves largely believe in the idea that supporting the state is the best way for "Asian nations to develop" and the most sustainable way to improve health services for women and children. With state distribution as JSA's central goal, Cambodian program managers understand themselves to be engaging in a "Japanese" or "Asian" (staff use the terms interchangeably) model of development. Program manager Boran explains, "It is the Japanese way for a strong state to upgrade the health services."

The second reason is that friendly relations with state officials also align with managers' personal career interests. Most program managers aspire to move into public health jobs later in their career, which will be discussed in more detail in later chapters. This means friendships with officials serve not only JSA's needs but managers' own professional goals. The third reason successful friendships are achievable is because of the friendly geopolitical relations between Cambodia and Japan. The Asian imaginary of state-led development does not resonate just with managers: it is being disseminated by political leaders in Cambodia, as we saw in the opening narrative of this chapter. Staff often employ the Asian imaginary to create and bolster relationships with officials. They describe the positive relationship between Cambodia and Japan as "Asian friendship." State partnership is also eased by JSA's commitment to the Cambodian Ministry of Health's policies and its ability to pay per diems. In consequence, JSA's managers build meaningful and personal connections with government officials when they find officials with the right power networks and willingness to cooperate.

The resonance of the distributor model and friendships between managers and public health officials has a positive impact on JSA's ability to implement technical workshops with its state partner. At JSA, in many cases, state officials actively participate in NGO trainings and meetings. In one workshop, Boran and Samnang spend three days discussing JSA's baseline data with Dr. Kim and two district health department officials. Together, the men examine findings on maternal nutrition, child nutrition, sanitation, maternal health center visits, and birthing practices. By the end of the workshop, Dr. Kim enthusiastically makes a presentation about JSA's data. On our lunch break, I ask Dr. Kim why he likes working with JSA. He reports he believes that JSA's programming is good for Cambodia because "their program and the MOH (Ministry of Health) policy are the same" and "Japan is a friend to Cambodia." At a later visit to his office, in a clear instance of inter-Asian referencing, Dr. Kim tells me that he likes the idea that Cambodia can have a health system like Thailand's. He believes aid from Japan can provide strong leadership to achieve that. He is proud to take part in creating that.

In interactions with government staff, all NGO workers must worry about how to "save face" as it is frowned upon to give direct advice or criticism to people who are superior to you in the Cambodian social hierarchy, like government officials. Friendly relationships allowed JSA program managers to engage in informal conversations about health education, though managers were careful to defer to officials' authority. For instance, in meetings like the one above, Samnang always asks Dr. Kim questions that defer to his expertise on topics such as how to improve the diversity of food groups eaten by pregnant women. However, cordial conversations allowed JSA staff to politely float new ideas and information to provincial and district officials.

At the baseline data workshop above, Dr. Kim was practicing his presentation on JSA's health data because he will make this presentation at the provincial and then national maternal and child health conferences in the next few months. Dr. Kim is grateful to JSA's managers for assisting him, and these men frequently have drinks together. This would not happen at USFA, where data is publicly presented by USFA staff and carefully branded with USAID/USFA logos. When I ask Samnang why he will not be presenting the data at the national conference himself, he says what his group does is "empower state officials to do this themselves, to implement their own policies." This is a very different notion of the "who" and "how" of empowerment than we find in U.S. INGOs, and one that resonates with public health partners.

The distributor model is reinforced by both Cambodian managers and state officials. This means that JSA is able to succeed in upgrading the skills of public health staff, at least to some degree, as officials actively engage in JSA's workshops. Due to this, JSA's partnership does assist the public health workers in the goal of distributing health services to all Cambodian women, regardless of class status. In this case, the imaginary of the "Asian way" is used to improve Cambodian women's lives by upgrading public maternal health services.

However, it must be noted, despite JSA's successes, it is unclear whether implementation will continue once JSA is no longer at least partially supporting the health education and services. Sovann expresses this concern to me: "We try to find the most committed officials . . . but it is not easy . . . and once the money is gone you don't always know what they will do." JSA staff gently advocate for officials to direct their budget towards these services, but only time will tell if JSA's state-as-distributor model is able to create sustainable changes in public health services. Nevertheless, like Dr. Kim above, after working with JSA, many public health officials expressed a desire to provide all women and children with improved public health services, often mentioning other Asian healthcare models like those of Thailand, South Korea, or Japan.

CO-OPTATION AND MASCULINE AUTHORITY

However, while JSA's partnership may improve women's public healthcare access, it does so through the reinforcement of the public health sector as a masculinized workplace (Vong et al. 2019). Although the share of female entry-level public health staff is increasing, men continue to dominate the leadership positions in the Cambodian public health system. The system is also highly centralized and hierarchical, meaning those in positions of power have great influence over the staff they oversee (Frieson et al. 2011; Johnson 2018). Additionally, 84 percent of Cambodian medical doctors are male, creating a near gender monopoly on medical knowledge (Khim et al. 2020). As JSA hires largely male program managers to interface with largely male public health officials, it creates a masculinized workplace within its own organization and partnership. This ends up enabling the use of the Asian imaginary to reinforce masculine authority in the public health sector.

One day, I travel with Samnang and Boran to visit Dr. Kim at his office. The three men discuss why pregnant women lack diversity in their diet.

They consider access to particular food groups, such as legumes, and financial barriers. However, both Dr. Kim and Boran agree that one of the most important issues is women's "low" health knowledge. Rural women, who are frequently portrayed as "poor and backwards," are frequently targets of domestic and international development agendas, and JSA is no exception (Puri 2003). Boran states, "the village mothers, the village health volunteers, and the midwives lack knowledge. They need to listen to us, their doctors, and health center workers [who are frequently men] to improve their diet." In conversations like these, women's limited knowledge is typically determined by men to be the largest barrier to improving maternal and child health, ignoring factors like financial constraints or resistant husbands.

After the meeting, I am dropped off at the provincial health department's small, open-air library above the courtyard since a woman, even a foreigner, does not need to be involved in male bonding rituals. Boran and Samnang head to the courtyard of the health department to play Ping-Pong with the vice provincial health director, as part of an effort to bolster their relationships with provincial officials. Over the game, I listen to them discuss their role in creating a strong public health system like Thailand's. All the women who work at the health department are also notably absent from this game.

Khmer managers weave male authority in public health positions into the Asian imaginary. Boran invites provincial and district health department staff to join him at a café, where we drink coffee and watch films. In this area, only men frequent this type of coffee shop, and thus, only male officials feel comfortable attending the meeting. I sit with the group and put my feet up to watch the film, eliciting laughs from the group that a woman is in this space. The men discuss how to improve the knowledge of mothers and female village health volunteers. When I ask Boran why he held the meeting at that type of café, he explains quite explicitly that he wanted to get to know male public health officials in a comfortable environment. He explains I might not "get it," since the West is all about formal meetings, but this is how "we" work in Asia.

The Cambodian public health system is a male-dominated space. Managers use the Asian imaginary alongside JSA's state-as-distributor model to explicitly reinforce the hierarchical public health system, with men at the top and male medical authority over women's bodies. In consequence, the outcome of JSA's partnership with the Cambodian public health system is not black and white. It succeeds in reinforcing donor intentions for the state-as-distributor model to upgrade publicly available and affordable health services for all mothers, regardless of class status. However, it is also co-opted to reinforce the public health sector as a masculinized workplace. Cambodian managers and state officials work together to craft their own vision of an "Asian" state in which men are the political leaders, but there is universal access to public healthcare (Connell 1990).

U.S. Family Aid: The State-as-Coordinator Model

In a staff meeting, practitioners sit around a conference table in U.S. Family Aid's (USFA) large, air-conditioned multistory office, located in one of the wealthier neighborhoods in Phnom Penh. Again, staff discuss successful cooperation with their government partner. However, USFA's government partner is not a provincial health department but instead a national sub-agency under the Ministry of Health, which I call the Cambodian Center for Health Communication (or the Center).

USFA aims to assist the Center in creating a coordination system or clearinghouse within their agency. The idea is that Center staff will monitor private and nonprofit health actors implementing health education activities in Cambodia. USFA's director, Ranny, explains to staff that they need to help the Center monitor the healthcare sector. In the end, USFA's goal for its state partnership is to illustrate how useful the Center's coordination system is and then advocate with the Ministry of Health for continued funding to sustain it after USAID funding ends. This is a very different role for the state than we saw at JSA. USFA's main objectives include implementing health behavior change programs in its target areas through supporting nonprofits and private clinics as well as "strengthening the co-ordination role of the public sector." In this model, the state has more of a facilitative role, in which it will monitor private and nonprofit actors, which I call *the state-as-coordinator* model.

The state-as-coordinator model reflects the U.S. healthcare system and its residual welfare policies in which the state plays a limited role. The health system in the U.S. is disjointed and complex due to distinct policies passed at different points in history. It relies heavily on private and nonprofit actors for service provision; and public healthcare provisions are given to the elderly or means-tested benefits to the poor, which are currently facing cuts (Dorn 2025; Quadagno 2010; Stevens 2008). Consequently, in Washington, D.C., several INGO and donor interviewees often describe the market as the primary solution to social issues, with INGOs and the state filling in gaps where the market fails.

Donors, specifically those from the U.S., Australia, and many nations in Europe, historically preferred to work with nongovernmental actors over unreliable country governments (Packard 2016). This funding trend has recently been challenged with the promotion of universal healthcare through the UN's Sustainable Development Goals discussed above. In consequence, engaging the state in healthcare has increased in U.S. INGOs, but it still takes place alongside the assumption that the market will be a key distributor of health services and nonprofits, and the state will fill in gaps. In Washington, D.C., one INGO interviewee explains their work with an initiative in Cambodia called ID Poor, which tries to subsidize public healthcare for the poorest citizens in the country. For this interviewee, if the government can help just these people, everyone else can purchase healthcare. Such beliefs illustrate that the assumption in the U.S. is that healthcare provision should not be solely in the hands of the public sector.

Consequently, in the state-as-coordinator model, the U.S. gender regime displays two assumptions about the public health system and women's healthcare. First, it promotes women's ability to consume healthcare, purchasing it from private clinics or receiving it from nonprofit actors. Second, it assumes only the poorest women will need to seek maternal and reproductive healthcare services through the public sector.

PARTNER AGENCY SELECTION

When I ask USFA's director, Ranny, why USFA works with the Cambodia Center for Health Communication, she explains that in the request for grant applications, the Center was identified by USAID as a strong candidate for coordinating organizations implementing health behavior change[6] activities. The Center is a national health subagency with limited political influence within the Ministry of Health, but it does have a history of working with international donors. Ranny believes the partnership is due to historic relationships. USFA's health project works to revitalize a 2015 World Health Organization program that supported the Center as a health education coordinator.

Yet, the Center's history with international donors has unexpected consequences for the partnership. One day, at a workshop, the facilitator inquires why the Center was originally created. An older Center staff member reflects on the health agency's origins. The Ministry of Health founded the subunit in 1994. The Center was created for public education and disease prevention projects, a topic that international donors and INGOs were providing funding to implement. While not said at the meeting, it must also be noted that the Center originated during the period when the ruling parties created several government agencies to increase client-patron networks, rewarding the politically loyal with government positions (Un 2005).

The official proudly notes that, over the years, the Center has worked on numerous media campaigns such as tuberculosis, HIV/AIDs prevention, smoking cessation, hygiene, and so on. Such campaigns are largely funded by international donors like the UN and World Health Organization. Thus, the Center was deemed the best candidate for this coordination role, perhaps because it is a more "civil society–like" government unit. A large percentage of the Center's funding comes from international donors, it plays an extremely limited role in health policy construction, and it competes with other health subagencies, such as National Center for Maternal and Child Health or the National Center for Tuberculosis, for funding from international donors. At the outset of the project, USAID and USFA may have assumed this situation would allow them to have more influence over the Center and its activities.

Following a U.S. gender regime, USFA works to assist the Center to regulate health education services for women and their families provided by private and nonprofit healthcare actors, assuming a hybrid healthcare system as the ideal model. This could indeed be a useful role for the Center to play. Cambodia has an enormous number of international and local NGOs implementing varied health behavior change projects as well as numerous unmonitored private clinics in its cities and provincial towns. If one government institution could monitor all of these activities, standardize health education and services, and let NGOs or private clinics know where services were needed, it could make nonstate healthcare more effective. Yet, as we will see below, this model does not resonate with Cambodian practitioners or state officials.

PROJECT ACTIVITIES

USFA's work to encourage the Center's staff to enact a coordination role occurs via numerous workshops. Workshops cover topics like marketing the Center as a health behavior change coordination agency, the Center's organizational effectiveness, the Center's financial advocacy, designing a health behavior change handbook for the Center to disperse, and setting up a health behavior change database housed in the Center. International experts are often hired to conduct these workshops.

One marketing workshop was centered around helping the Center "create a marketing campaign" to "brand themselves" as the health behavior change experts in Cambodia. It was facilitated by a leader from a private marketing firm that USFA has partnered with for this USAID project. An energetic German woman, Brigette, is flown in to facilitate the event. Brigette lets us know she will be using the up-to-date tools of "human-centered design"[7] to analyze the Center's needs and "solve their problem." To begin, she provides Center officials in attendance with data she and her staff collected about the current lack of knowledge on the Center's role in provincial health offices and other government subunits. Then she informs Center staff that she can help them position their organization as "the expert in Cambodian health behavior change."

Brigette asks Center staff to estimate how much time per month they can spend on coordinating nonstate health actors. By this point, the Center's director, who has been perusing the data that Brigette offered, seems annoyed. First, he questions the data—"Who did your staff interview?" "Where did you ask people these questions?" "Are you suggesting that the Cambodian people think the Center's current work is not important?" Then he addresses the topic of the new coordination role supported by USFA. He inquires why USFA does not want the Center itself to do a campaign on health behavior change and women's health. Then he asserts energetically that "we [the Center staff] have our roles in the ministry to worry about, we have no free time to approve NGOs, private clinics, or other subunits' work; my staff needs to be paid more if you are going to bring more work." He pointedly asks Brigette, Why does she "bring more work but not more budget?" Unlike JICA, which provides per diems, USAID has strict rules against paying government officials, and Center staff do not receive per diem for attending USFA's workshops, much less payment for coordination activities.

Brigette pivots, enthusiastically stating that they should move on to a discussion of how the Center can set itself up to get paid for its coordinator role. The Center's deputy director cuts her off, explaining that they already tried this with the previous World Health Organization project; the Ministry of Health does not condone taking money for coordinating projects. He says the World Health Organization was informed of this during the previous project and its representatives talked to the Ministry of Health about the issue, but nothing changed. He starts discussing possible workarounds, like taking per diem from NGOs to support the Center's coordinating work, at which point Brigette looks to USFA's director, Ranny, for help.

Ranny jumps into the conversation, speaking initially in the workshop language of English and then switching to Khmer. She is respectful, calculated, and convincing with her words. She explains she is just an NGO director, and one NGO does not have the power to coordinate all the different nonstate actors. She is aware the Center was not created to coordinate NGOs or private clinics, but there is a real need for it. She carefully rationalizes the project activities, telling Center staff that if the entire country had consistent and coordinated health behavior change programming, the implementation of health services by nongovernment actors would be far more effective. In her opinion, the Ministry of Health has the money to cover this activity, but it needs to see its usefulness first. If the Center shows the Ministry of Health how effective it is in coordination, perhaps it will be able to carve out a permanent funding niche for itself in the ministry's budget. She finishes speaking by noting that, of course, this is the Center's decision, as they are the government officials. Despite Ranny's words, the Center's deputy director continues to insist that the ministry will never fund such activities and asks why USAID does not fund the Center to provide health education directly. Such disagreements over the feasibility of the coordination role were not uncommon.

Outside of large workshops, USFA staff also have periodic smaller meetings with the Center leaders. There, USFA tries to get the Center's "input" or "approval" on the implementation of health education aspects of its project, something USAID encourages. However, these meetings are not always regarded as useful. After returning from a meeting on health behavior change messaging, USFA's monitoring and evaluation specialist, Panh, informs me it is difficult to get the Center staff to make decisions; they do not provide useful input, and it is increasingly challenging to get attendance from higher-level staff.

In addition, in the U.S.-funded aid chain, state cooperation takes place at two levels: the national level in USFA's work with the Center as well as through USFA's local NGO subgrantees. Since JSA implements through the state directly, it does not subgrant to local nonprofit partners. In contrast, USFA funds local NGOs, like the subgrantee which I observed, the Cambodian Development Society (CDS), to directly implement health education and services for women. CDS's main focus is implementing health education programming in rural communities. But, as CDS's director explains, to implement its projects the organization "carefully cooperates" with local state officials, including district health centers, commune councils, and village chiefs, informing them of activities, asking for their advice on specific needs in the area, and attending NGO meetings coordinated by local government offices.

In reality, this means CDS's state partnership is largely limited to brief meetings with local-level officials asking for input about where CDS's services are most needed. I observed this firsthand when I traveled with the manager of CDS's health team, Reasmey, to one of CDS's target communes. Before going to conduct village health trainings for mothers, we go to the commune office to talk with the deputy commune chief. After introducing herself, Reasmey carefully explains CDS's mission, what the project is about, how it will help women in the area (by preventing maternal death, a neutral and appealing goal), and asks for their "input." Formally, the deputy chief tells her that he believes decreasing maternal death is a worthy goal and describes a few villages that might need her attention. After gaining the "support" of the commune leaders, we head out, and she and her team members travel to multiple villages, conducting community trainings for women. When I ask Reasmey about the purpose of the preliminary meeting with the deputy chief, she informs me that for "government cooperation," we just need them to "know us and approve our plan so we don't get in trouble."

CDS illustrates two things about USFA's coordinator model. First, USFA's funding to nonprofit implementing partners like CDS further demonstrates its assumption that the government will be one among many health service distributors for women. Second, supporting USFA's goals, CDS allows the state to act as a coordinator of its activities, at least in a limited way, reinforcing USFA's vision of the state as coordinator.

U.S. Family Aid and Development Imaginaries: Busy Staff and Frustrated Officials

As the workshop above started to illustrate, at USFA, both state actors and practitioners resist the state-as-coordinator model. However, unlike at JSA, where practitioners and state officials work together, practitioners and officials resist the model for separate reasons. Cambodian staff resist by employing rhetoric about their commitment to the imaginary of the West. In contrast, state officials employ the Asian imaginary to reject the work of USFA.

RESISTANCE BY STAFF

At a staff meeting one day, we sit looking up at the project's current work-plan, which includes a detailed Excel spreadsheet of over a hundred activities USFA staff must complete in the next two years. After the meeting, the chief of party, Dr. Belinda, laments the difficulty of fulfilling all the project requirements. USFA needs to subgrant to and monitor local NGOs in implementing its health programs, enhance the quality of private clinics, and support the public health system in a coordination role. Throughout the meeting, she laments, "Why do we need to work with everyone?" "How can we do it all?"

In contrast to Japan Services Asia's (JSA) friendships with state officials, there is a lack of commitment on the part of USFA staff and sometimes open resistance to the state partnership. USFA staff resist the state-as-coordinator model for three reasons. First, practically speaking, staff oppose the model because they lack time for state partnership. As we have seen, USFA staff are required to engage with a substantially larger number of stakeholders than JSA staff.[8] Managing this larger number of activities, USFA's program staff do not have the same amount of time to devote to building strong relationships with government officials as the male managers hired specifically to engage in those relationships at JSA.

Second, staff resist USFA's state-as-coordinator goals, not just with complaints of limited time, but by arguing civil society organizations, like INGOs, are better suited to assist women and Cambodian communities. It does not hurt that, by upholding the need for INGOs, practitioners can ensure they keep their jobs. This resistance is often justified by rejecting the idea that working with the Cambodian state is a part of what a Western INGO should be doing. One USFA project director, Chanmony, complains that in the past "the Western donors wanted to support civil society because the Cambodian state cannot give the rural people, particularly the mothers in remote areas, what they need."

Another staff member argues that she thought Americans knew the Cambodian state is never going to pursue women's empowerment and that is why civil society needs to do this work. Staff employ the imaginary of the West and its support for civil society as the right way to improve women's health. Some even felt somewhat betrayed by the donor turn towards state partnership. Staff members are also deeply embedded in social networks with international donors, other NGOs, and private clinics (where they might get future jobs), and therefore they are less interested in building relationships with state officials.

Third, USFA faces tension due to the strained geopolitical relationship between Cambodia and the United States. Cambodian government officials expressed distaste for USFA's model and mistrust of USAID and the U.S. government more broadly. USFA staff feel the relationship between practitioners and Center officials is difficult because there is a distain for "Western intervention" among state officials. This tension is worsened by the fact that USAID does not allow USFA to pay officials per diem. Program manager Bopha argues with Ranny about this in a staff meeting one day. Bopha is asked to gather provincial- and national-level state officials for a workshop. She contests this stating, "You know it will never work!" She challenges Ranny, arguing that they cannot work with state officials successfully if USFA does not provide per diem.

In the face of time constraints, the valorization of the West as supporting civil society, and political tensions, state cooperation becomes more of a performative partnership for USFA employees. Staff see state cooperation as a donor-requirement box to check off by formally attending meetings and conducting the workshops as outlined in the workplan, in fact engaging with state partners in only a limited fashion.

Following suit, USFA's implementing subgrantee, Cambodian Development Society (CDS) staff also maintain a surface-level relationship with local officials and a commitment to the importance of civil society assistance for women. CDS's director, Rith, who founded CDS in the early 2000s, says that working with the state "is not so easy but not so bad." He acts as a "careful mediator." "I want the government to think we are there to help them, but also, I work with the grassroots people to improve the community voice. It is CDS's job to help the poor people, so we work between the government and the people. But we must be careful; they [government officials] cannot think we are raising the people against them or they will blacklist us." He goes on to explain that he was previously a monk, so it often helps him to ground his desire to help the poor in Buddhism, allowing him to present his work as apolitical and diminish apparent ties to the West.

According to CDS's women's health team director, Reasmey, securing government cooperation is the most difficult for community events, in which she needs to gather twenty to thirty community members for a family planning and maternal health training. She must take special precautions to get permissions from commune and village leaders, so her event is not misconstrued as mobilizing villagers. In the community event I attended, CDS staff provided resources for women to seek services from nearby private clinics or CDS itself. Village health volunteers and government officials played no role in the training, outside of providing permissions.

In its limited state interactions, CDS allows the state to act as coordinator, advising on where it implements activities, which allows CDS to keep donors and state officials alike happy. However, like USFA, the health team's partnership with the Cambodian state is fulfilled in a way that is, again, limited and assumes NGOs and private clinics will provide women with health services and education.

RESISTANCE BY STATE ACTORS

One day, at an organizational analysis workshop, Center staff are asked to identify their organization's goals for the future. Next, Center staff are broken into small groups to discuss different goals, which are written on posters in different areas of the conference room. One of these goals is financial sustainability. The workshop facilitator, an INGO employee from Eastern Europe, has already written possible subheadings on the financial sustainability poster, including budget advocacy at the Ministry of Health, resource mobilization strategy, and branding/marketing strategy.

When it comes time for the group that discussed financial sustainability to present its poster, it does not go the way USFA staff hoped. For the Center staff, budget advocacy has a different meaning. While they were tasked with discussing how to secure funds from the Ministry of Health or market their organization, they cross out Ministry of Health entirely and write "advocate for funding from donors like USAID, UNICEF, EU, UN, and UNFPA." They plan to use such funds so the Center can implement its own health education campaigns. For Center officials, the coordinator model envisioned by USFA is not legitimated in the goals, policies, and funding structures of the Ministry of Health.

Unlike USFA staff, who emphasize civil society organizations as distributors of health services, state officials reject the idea that the state should be a coordinator for a different reason. They argue the Center itself should be the distributor of health education, not NGOs. Center officials often complain that USFA is just part of the problem with "Western nations intervening" in the work of the Cambodian government. At a workshop, the Center manager I sit next to points out, "Why would we want to be like the U.S.? Healthcare is so expensive there!" She goes on to tell me that she thinks the Cambodian Ministry of Health should follow the strong model of Thailand's successful public healthcare. Many Center officials expressed the belief that foreign donors should provide the funding directly to the Cambodian state, which would then distribute health services and education.

At another workshop, I share my table with a Center staff member who has worked for the agency since the 1990s. As the meeting nears a close, she inquires when USFA will provide the Center with the computers, server, and technical assistance outlined in the project documents. She gruffly reports USFA is asking Center staff to come to endless workshops and meetings, but she is tired of talk. She is beginning to wonder if she can trust USFA to provide the computers. She goes on to explain that the coordinator role will not work. It is just "talk" and "MOH [Ministry of Health] will not provide funds to the Center for talk."

She further proclaims that "women deserve these services directly from us" and the Center requires donor support to conduct its work, "that is how we do things." The Center engages in the partnership with USFA for the benefits it will receive. At the same time, not unlike the official's speech at the beginning of this chapter, Center officials reinforce the Asian imaginary and disparage the West as "intervening." They argue donors should be supporting the Cambodian health sector in directly providing women's health services, not cultivating the private sector or NGOs. Thus, USFA's state-as-coordinator model, and its inherent assumption that women should be enabled to consume healthcare services through the private and nonprofit sector, is actively resisted by government officials at the Center.

Implementer-Distributor Model Interactions

It should be clear by now that Cambodian practitioners are aware of both JSA's state-as-distributor model and USFA's state-as-coordinator model. Practitioners compare the two models to one another and integrate them into their imaginaries of development in the West and Asia. However, Japanese practitioners in Tokyo and Cambodia also engage in inter-Asian comparisons of public health systems and developmental states. One day at lunch, Junko tells me about a fish we're eating. She explains that this fish is called "the Japanese fish" in Khmer because it was supposedly given to Cambodia long ago by a Japanese emperor. She states, "even in that time, the Japanese were helping to improve the health of their smaller neighbor kingdom." In this way, she positions Japan as a powerful, paternal figure to Southeast Asian nations.

Junko also went to graduate school in Thailand and admires the Thai health system. She encourages her managers' belief that, with Japan's support, the Cambodian health system can become more like Thailand's. However, when I ask her about JSA's limited support for private health clinics, she laughs. Junko tells me that everyone but the Americans knows the public health system should be primary.

Similarly, in Tokyo, there is a strong belief that promoting a strong state is the "Asian" way, but inter-Asian comparisons are made to discuss how Japan can distinguish itself. At a conference about aid to Africa in Tokyo, there were several discussions about how, while both Japan and China support strong states, Japanese aid needs to "differentiate itself" from Chinese aid. One representative from Japan's Ministry of Foreign Affairs describes Japan as the "only non-Western democratic leader giving aid to Africa, so Africa can learn from us how to make a strong state."[9] He goes on to restate the importance of Japan strategically posing itself as an alternative to China and to the West in its aid to Africa.

In contrast, when asked about an Asian development model, most American interviewees in Phnom Penh and Washington, D.C., had limited knowledge about Asian donors. Some practitioners from the U.S. in Phnom Penh are aware, to some degree, of the work of JICA or KOICA (South Korea's bilateral agency), but comment that those donors are small or keep to themselves. Practitioners frequently remark on the lack of "political work" done by Asian nations. One interviewee in Washington, D.C., says she believes JICA engages in largely depoliticized projects in infrastructure, health, and education. "Yeah, it's [those sectors are] just safe . . . that just seems to be like the low-hanging fruit whereas we do actual work."

Similarly, an American USFA headquarters staff member tells me that when she was a Peace Corps volunteer, she met several JICA and KOICA volunteers. She found them "sketchy" as they all worked within government ministries, all they cared about was state relationships, and they seemed to be "funneling money or something." Finally, if China came up, the general sentiment of American practitioners is "don't get me started" on the problems with China's aid model. Practitioners frequently commented that

Chinese loans are simply going to further indebt the Global South (with no acknowledgment of the fact that U.S.-led organizations like the World Bank and IMF have also been giving out loans for decades).

This finding that American practitioners disparage the Asian development model aligns with other studies that document how, in the West, Asian donors, and their cooperation with recipient state officials, are often associated with "cronyism" and "corruption" to delegitimize their work (Hall 2003). Yet, as this chapter has illustrated, while Japanese INGOs do work closely with developing states, this does not necessarily mean their work should be immediately assumed to be ineffective or corrupt.

The Cambodian State's Turn Towards Asia

To conclude this chapter, I will examine two interrelated questions about the outcomes of JSA's and USFA's state partnerships. What effect might each INGO have on the Cambodian state's capacity? And what benefits or limitations does each INGO partnership have for the state's impact on women's health outcomes? In JSA's case, state actors and Cambodian managers work together to use the Asian imaginary to implement a strong public health model. In the long run, this could increase state capacity to provide maternal healthcare services to all women, particularly those in poor and rural areas. In this way, the imaginary of strong Asian states is utilized to upgrade women's lives. Yet, at the same time, JSA's preference for hiring male managers who can interface smoothly with high-ranking male state officials creates a deeply masculinized workplace. Consequently, state actors and JSA's managers use the idea of a strong Asian state to reinforce male medical authority in the public health system. Here we see the contradictory outcomes the Asian imaginary can have when it comes to improving Cambodian women's lives.

At USFA, staff use the imaginary of the West and civil society to resist state partnership, spending as little time as possible engaging state officials at the Cambodian Center for Health Communication. In this case, the notion that INGOs funded by the U.S., Australia, and Europe should be civil society actors that empower women is used in a way that does not immediately help to improve women's access to health services. USFA practitioners resist investing time and energy into helping state actors coordinate NGO and private health services.

In contrast to USFA workers, state officials that work with USFA reject the West and embrace the Asian imaginary of strong public health systems to resist USFA's state-as-coordinator model. In consequence, USFA's model does little to change state actor capacity. The significance of this for Cambodian women's health is not cut and dried. On the one hand, we can imagine that in another recipient nation, a developing state actively working to regulate the private sector could upgrade services provided to women in private clinics. Yet Cambodian officials are not wrong to be skeptical of the U.S. healthcare model. The U.S. spends more on healthcare than any other industrialized nation but does not have considerably better health outcomes to show for it (Gunja, Gumas, and Williams 2023). Nations in the Global South increasingly advocate that public healthcare funding is the better path to achieve the long-term goal of universal healthcare. So it is also possible the Center officials may benefit women's health provision in the long run by rejecting the U.S. hybrid healthcare model.

In each INGO case, what Cambodian practitioners and state officials decide to do in response to donor activities is what dictates the outcome of each partnership. To return to the official's speech from the beginning of the chapter, it is clear a strong "Asian" public health system is appealing to state actors across the board. In turning towards Asia, Cambodian public health officials imagine themselves following in the footsteps of other nations in their region. In this way, Cambodian state actors challenge long-held Western neoliberal development agendas that promote retrenchment and privatization of state services. Moreover, through different uses of the imaginaries in this chapter we start to see something that will become increasingly clear through the chapters of this book. It is not possible to simply say that the development imaginary of the West empowers women while the Asian imaginary does not. Development imaginaries have diverse impacts on INGO practitioner implementation, modification, or resistance. This will become even clearer in the next chapter, which analyzes the implementation process for each INGO's women's health activities.

In conclusion, this chapter illustrates that to understand an INGO's ability to upgrade state capacity, it is essential to examine two aspects of INGO-state partnerships. First, we must look at how an INGO's donor's priorities and gender regime shape interactions with a recipient nation. While JSA and USFA both engage in partnerships with public health agencies, donor gender regimes impact the partnerships each INGO pursues. If the Cambodian health system is a puzzle, with INGO services filling in certain missing pieces, the pieces funded by Japan and the U.S. are dissimilar shapes. Second, the outcomes of partnerships are also determined by whether an INGO's goals resonate with INGO practitioners and the recipient state partners. If INGOs want to effectively intervene in the work of governing and social service provision, they must attend to the degree to which their partnership goals are legitimate in the eyes of the recipient state.

THREE

"Modern Asian Mothers" or "Empowered Consumers"?
Imaginations of Modernity and Tradition

The Cambodian government's celebration for National Maternal and Child Health Day is held at a large riverside hotel in Phnom Penh. Its funders—the United Nations, the German bilateral agency GIZ, and USAID—pulled out all the stops for this celebration. I sit in the audience with at least two hundred representatives from NGOs, private clinics, public health workers, and midwives in training. A USAID-funded women's health NGO has been tasked with performing an educational skit about infant health and family planning. Such a skit is an example of one that would be used by NGOs to educate villagers in rural Cambodia.

We watch as one male and two female actors come onto the stage decked out in sparkling, traditional-style Cambodian clothing. The audience giggles as one woman tries to incorrectly feed, clothe, and hold a plastic newborn. Slapstick comedy ensues around the female actor's inability to care for the plastic baby. The other two actors crack jokes as they educate her about feeding times, the necessity of health checkups for mom and baby, and infant nutrition. Then she shyly asks about preventing the next baby from coming too soon, which incites laughter from the audience. The female actor educates her about family planning, explaining the different birth control methods. Then the male actor says, he knows it is embarrassing, but both the husband and wife need to be knowledgeable on this topic. Yet he also asserts that it is okay to feel shy about discussing family planning. "Asians do not talk so loudly about such things like foreigners . . . in Cambodia it is new for men and women to talk about family planning together."

In this skit, we again see the use of imaginaries differentiating Asia from the West, but this time in the implementation of women's health education. This chapter delves into what Japan Services Asia and U.S. Family Aid's women's health projects *actually do* for women in Cambodia. Each INGO works to upgrade women's health services in rural areas, and, in doing so, provides some form of health education. However, the education and services they provide are different. As we saw in the previous chapter, the gender regimes of the U.S. and Japan prioritize different women's health needs. Japanese staff at Japan Services Asia describe their maternal health project as helping women become educated about maternal and child health and how to access effective public health services, creating "modern Asian mothers." In contrast, staff at U.S. Family Aid implement activities that provide maternal and reproductive health services through the private and nonprofit sector, envisioning women as "empowered consumers."

Khmer practitioners interpret each donor's distinctive women's health project activities through the development imaginaries, as we saw NGO practitioners do in the skit above. In doing so, practitioners in both INGOs modify the health education and services received by beneficiaries in rural Cambodia. However, before presenting these findings, I investigate how the concepts of "traditional" and "modern" have historically been used to describe gender relations in Cambodia. These concepts play a key role in practitioners' discussions about how to implement development activities.

"Traditional" and "Modern" Women in Cambodia

Beliefs about gender and family relations are often at the heart of debates around what it would mean for a nation to become modern while maintaining its unique cultural traditions. Gender and family dynamics are key sites of global development activities aimed to upgrade societies and recipient-nation adaptations (Davis 2007; Suh 2021; Tavory and Swidler 2009; Vijayakumar 2021). Yet the critiques of women, and sometimes men, as being "too modern" and abandoning a nation's cultural traditions that are levied in many discussions of international development today are not new. Such critiques became prominent in many postcolonial countries during anticolonial and nationalist struggles. Nationalist groups constructed idealized visions of their nation's cultural traditions and the place of women and families in them. They did so to push back on the Western other and ensure their nation did not get swallowed up in what they saw as the homogenizing forces of modernization (Jacobsen 2008; Narayan 1997). Following this trend, in Cambodia, debates about the role of gender and tradition in Cambodia's modernity have been prominent since the postcolonial era.

Cambodia gained independence from France and Norodom Sihanouk took power in 1953. To reestablish cultural traditions of the past, Sihanouk and the political elites of the time looked to the recent past. Just before the colonial period began in 1863, Cambodia was ruled by King Ang Duong, who won independence from the Vietnamese in 1848. Despite many historical instances of a social order with more egalitarian gender roles in Cambodia, during Ang Duong's reign, Cambodia was in a moment of gender backlash due to several factors. These included the assumption that it was their previous queen's fault Cambodia was colonized by the Vietnamese (despite it largely being her father that sold Cambodia to Vietnam) and the influence of the nearby Thai court, where Buddhist principles that associated women with "ignoble behavior" were circulating. Additionally, the French conjectured that Cambodian women were "sexually debaucherous" and in need of civilizing (Jacobsen 2008). French rulers then pushed women out of many positions of power in Cambodia during colonization, thus limiting women's ability to influence the construction of gendered cultural traditions in the Sihanouk era.

This meant that when Sihanouk came to power, he looked to cultural documents written in Ang Duong's time, such as the Cbpab Srei (Code for women). The Cbpab Srei is a Khmer poem and female code of conduct. This code was written for and read only by nobles in Ang Doung's time but is now taught in Cambodian public schools today. It compares girls to cloth, whose virtue is easily soiled by sexual promiscuity, while boys are likened to gold (Anderson and Grace 2018). The poem goes on to prescribe that women should be quiet and submissive towards their husbands as well as the primary keepers of home and children (Brickell 2011). In the Sihanouk era, "people perceived gender roles in traditional Cambodian society to reflect those outlined in the Cbpab Srei, without reflecting upon the possible biases and motivations of its authors and dismissing other evidence of egalitarianism or status for women in Cambodian rural traditions, because they were those of socially insignificant people rather than the elite" (Jacobsen 2008: 171). Reconstruction of the "traditional" cultural roles of women played an important role in Cambodia's postcolonial nationalist narrative until Sihanouk lost power in 1970.

Similarly, after the Khmer Rouge period, and the long civil war that followed it, when Cambodia reconstructed its society in the early 1990s, it again returned to the traditions promoted in the Ang Duong and Sihanouk eras. Belief systems that contend men are higher on the status hierarchy than women were reinstated alongside "traditional" forms of patronage and nepotism. Political elites promoted the idea that if women took up their "traditional" roles, they would protect Cambodian culture and restore the nation. Yet, also in the 1990s, Cambodia saw an influx of international rhetoric around gender equality. This rhetoric was coming from the United Nations, which was assisting with the establishment of democracy in the country at this time, alongside the many international development organizations that came to assist the UN (Jacobsen 2008).

With the rise in foreign aid funding, a massive number of women's NGOs were founded in Cambodia throughout the 1990s and early 2000s. These organizations promote women's empowerment activities and trainings throughout Cambodia (Jacobsen 2010). Under the guidance of Western donors, many of these organizations blame traditional Cambodian cultural beliefs as a key cause of some gender inequities in the country, like violence against women. Such accusations only furthered the assumption that feminism was a foreign import that was undermining Cambodian cultural traditions. In consequence, presently there are multiple, sometimes conflicting beliefs about femininity and masculinity, and what makes a "modern" or "traditional" man or woman in Cambodian society.

These various gendered beliefs come to the surface when development practitioners attempt to implement projects that will advance women's lives, families, and health. This chapter finds competing Asian and Western development imaginaries are the battlefront on which "traditional" and "modern" gendered beliefs are reinforced, hybridized, and contested. As development and gender relations are not natural givens, but instead historical and social constructions, in making these arguments, practitioners play a part in reconstructing the role of gender and family in Cambodia's national advancement.

Japan Services Asia: "Modern Asian Mothers"
WOMEN'S HEALTH AND JAPAN'S GENDER REGIME

As discussed in chapter 2, Japanese donor and headquarter organizations emphasize the need to support maternal and child health programs that foster an effective public health system. The design of these projects is impacted by Japan's successful legacy of maternal healthcare, its own history of family planning services, and the decision to largely ignore global gender equality rhetoric.

JICA documents and interviewees report that their aid directly attempts to export Japan's own great success in improving maternal and child health outcomes. After World War II, Japan was plagued by high infant and maternal death rates. Yet today its infant and maternal mortality rates are some of the lowest in the world (Knoema 2018; Takeuchi, Sakagami, and Perez 2016). Japan's rapid decrease in its infant and maternal mortality rates is attributed to high government investment, including training and deployment of public midwives and nurses, building maternal and child health centers, and the dispersal of Japan's Maternal and Child Health Handbook (JICA 2005; Takeuchi, Sakagami, and Perez 2016). The handbook, which began to be officially used all over the nation in 1947, provides both educational information to new mothers and record-keeping for maternal and infant health markers (Homei 2006; Takeuchi, Sakagami, and Perez 2016). Currently, the Japanese government provides free prenatal visits and a reimbursement allowance covering a large percentage of the cost of birth and delivery.

Maternal and infant health holds an important place in Japan's vision of its own modernization (Homei 2006; Takeuchi, Sakagami, and Perez 2016). As we saw earlier, Japanese INGOs are encouraged to promote Japan's maternal and infant healthcare model abroad. This includes the use of the Maternal and Child Health Handbook, supporting public health workers in rural communities, and promoting the improvement of health infrastructure. Additionally, Japanese health aid pushes countries in the Global South to move away from traditional health practices in favor of "modern" medicine. At a JICA-funded workshop for visiting public health officials from Africa, I observed a Japanese trainer provide attendees with detailed information about maternal and child health needs. Then she juxtaposed biomedical health practices with "traditional medicine models" that are dangerous for mothers. Attendees swap stories of the "crazy aunties and grandmothers" committed to traditional medicine. One official tells the story of an expectant grandmother who brought traditional herbs to the birthing center. The grandmother tried to give them to her daughter when the midwife was not looking. Attendees and the Japanese trainer laughed at her foolishness.

However, when it comes to reproductive health, JICA's activities are more limited. Examples of family planning activities are fewer on JICA's public website. Where they do exist, they are typically combined with, and take a backseat to, maternal health activities. When asked about family planning, one JICA interviewee reports, "well we do not often work on that health topic directly." This also comes out of Japan's own legacy of reproductive health politics.

In 1936, a Japanese woman named Shidzue Kato, a friend of Margaret Sanger, opened her first Birth Control Consultation Center in Tokyo, facing political repression at the time (Kato 1984). The Japanese government's emphasis on fertility in war time largely thwarted her efforts. The birth control pill was not approved for use in Japan until 1999, making Japan the last industrialized nation to legalize it. There is limited availability of medical contraception and a lack of education on contraceptive options in Japan. In Japan, 80 percent of married women rely on condoms and only 3 percent of women between the ages of sixteen and forty-nine report taking oral contraceptives (Htun 2013; Yoshida et al. 2016). As the country still struggles with low birthrates, it is not eager to encourage access to contraception. Subsequently, Japan also provides aid for very few family planning activities in the Global South.

Finally, in contrast to practitioners in Washington, D.C., donors and INGO headquarters staff in Tokyo contend that activities directly advocating against gender inequality are something Japanese aid should not do. Interviewees often explain that Japan does not wish to "intervene in other cultures" as aid donors from the West do. Yet, in Tokyo, it is implicitly assumed mothers will be the main caretakers of their own and their children's health. There is little to no discussion of fathers. For donor and INGO interviewees in Tokyo, advancing women's place in society will take place through enabling mothers to gain health knowledge as well as access to affordable, quality public maternal health services.

WOMEN'S HEALTH ACTIVITIES AT JAPAN SERVICES ASIA

Consequently, JSA's project activities emphasize, first, upgrading the capacity of public health officials, and next, educating mothers living in rural areas about maternal and infant health. JSA imparts scientific knowledge about maternal and child health by implementing its project through the "training the trainers" model discussed in chapter 2.

For example, JSA staff work with provincial officials to train district officials. One day, we go to the provincial hospital to meet the provincial director of maternal and child health, Dr. Kim, to do a training with two district health officials, Dr. Mao and Ms. Channy. There we rehearse for the health education workshop for the next level of training with health center workers. Using a flipbook with pictures of different stages of pregnancy and photos of different foods, Dr. Kim lectures on proper nutrition for newborns, pregnant women, and new mothers. He explains basic food groups, what pregnant women should eat, and the risk of anemia. He also details how long breastfeeding should last, what foods children need to eat from six months to two years of age, and when mothers should seek healthcare for their infants.

After coaching from Dr. Kim and JSA staff, Dr. Mao provides information on the frequency of healthcare visits expected during and after pregnancy as well as the importance of health center delivery. Then, he turns it over to Ms. Channy, who describes in detail how to breastfeed and how to cook *baw-baw grung*, a healthy meal of rice porridge and vegetables for babies. Ms. Channy and Dr. Mao receive updated health data and advice on their presentation from JSA staff and Dr. Kim. JSA's manager, Boran, explains to the health officials why using the Maternal and Child Health Handbook will allow Cambodian mothers to advance as Japan's mothers did.

After the workshops for provincial and district health staff, JSA supports a workshop for health center and commune officials. Dr. Kim and Dr. Mao present the health education trainings rehearsed in the previous workshop. At the end of the workshop, Ms. Channy facilitates as participants practice cooking *baw-baw grung* in small groups. Each group gets ingredients and a single gas stovetop. Male participants mostly sit or stand around, joking with one another. Older women take charge of each group, opening the recipe book, cooking the *baw-baw*, and younger women help chop and stir. Per JSA's agenda, biomedical information about maternal health and child nutrition is imparted at this workshop. Yet the process of dispersing the information is gendered. Male doctors provide scientific knowledge while Ms. Channy instructs participants on "women's issues" like breastfeeding and cooking. Then female participants do the cooking.

After this workshop, with the support of JSA staff, health center workers and commune officials train village health volunteers at multiple two-day workshops in different districts. At these workshops, health center workers, JSA male program managers, and district doctors again provide education on medical knowledge. Then female commune officials describe the process of breastfeeding and run the cooking training. At the final phase of the "training the trainers" process, JSA supports health center workers and village volunteers in leading multiple cooking trainings and health monitoring community events for pregnant women and the mothers of newborns in the villages.

At a village health monitoring event, about twenty new mothers or pregnant women are in attendance, waiting under the shade of the village's wooden meeting pavilion. We begin the training. Health center workers and JSA program assistants cajole babies onto the scale, speak to mothers, and record information on each woman and child, both in JSA's database and in each woman's JICA-branded Maternal and Child Health Handbook. Mothers of children who are underweight as well as pregnant women from the village who are not in attendance will receive home visits later that day.

As children are being measured, the JSA program manager in attendance, Samnang, and a health center worker coach the female village volunteer on what to say to the mothers, showing her the flipbook and quizzing her on appropriate diet and breastfeeding for children between six and eight months. She responds to their questions shyly, carefully calling both men *lou kru*, or "teacher," a title used to show respect in Cambodia. Once the training starts, the health volunteer nervously speaks on the topic of breastfeeding and nutrition, giggling and looking back at Samnang and the health center worker for approval. The men watch nearby as she goes through her information. After the ten-minute lecture the women all clap and cheer, congratulating her on completing the difficult task of speaking on scientific information.

While the data collected for this project focus on development practitioners, I did get some sense of beneficiary responses to each program by attending village trainings. Listening to beneficiary conversations during and after JSA's trainings, mothers have mixed responses. Waiting in line to receive soap after the completion of community events, mothers talk and laugh among themselves, sharing stories about the village, their children, or deliberating the marriage prospects of younger JSA program assistants who live nearby. One day, when discussing the training, a mother explains that her mother told her breastfeeding should be done for a different amount of time before giving solid food. Another village mother says she has heard babies should have water at times. The woman next to them shushes them and motions to Samnang and the health center worker, saying we must try to do what the *kru bat*, or medical professionals, say. Yet one mother scoffs at the training, saying it is a great idea to feed children all those nutritious foods, but who can afford it? And, if they did have the money, her husband would buy meat.

In response, a seasoned mother with a toddler and a newborn warns the debating women, you must keep up your child's weight like the book says, pointing to the Maternal and Child Health Handbooks each woman has been given. Otherwise, health center workers, JSA staff, and even district officials might come to your house and embarrass you in front of the village. Clearly, village women believe such house visits are a negative reflection on mothering skills and thus to be avoided. But, notably, while before and after they chat among themselves, during training, the women are largely silent.

Finally, village beneficiaries do not seem aware that JSA's funding comes from Japan, and neither do they engage with the development imaginaries. Instead, many focused on the individual practitioners from JSA and the assistance provided by them, evaluating them as possible patrons in the Cambodian patron-client system. Mothers tell stories about which JSA managers came to assist them, deliberate about whether JSA will provide their village with wells or livestock like other NGOs, and report to one another how close program assistants' families are in kinship ties to their village chief.

The Many Meanings of Asian Tradition: Reinforcement and Hybridization at Japan Services Asia

"For our country to advance, the pregnant woman must learn to eat healthy and listen to the modern doctor."
    —BORAN, JSA PROGRAM MANAGER

At JSA, practitioners use the development imaginary to both reinforce and hybridize donor intentions. First, JSA's managers advocate that it is "Asian tradition" for women to take on most of the work of childcare and household labor. However, Cambodian practitioners at JSA also modify JSA's health education to include "traditional" medicine.

REINFORCING "TRADITIONAL" GENDER ROLES

When I ask Boran which caregiver was interviewed during JSA's baseline survey, he looks confused, stating "in Cambodia, it is the mother who should take care of her child." Or, after I inquire why men are not invited to the village cooking trainings or health monitoring events, Sovann laughs, explaining these topics are "for the woman." Using Tokyo's noninterventionist stance when it comes to gender norms, JSA staff actively promote what they call "traditional Asian" household and family norms in project activities.

Only mothers attend community workshops; JSA does not address the need to educate male caretakers. At one village training, a village volunteer asks Sovann if she should recruit husbands to attend, and he tells her it is not necessary. In the view of Cambodian managers at JSA, a return to the traditional values of Asia, as opposed to Western norms for "gender equality," is what is needed in the "modern" world where Asia is a prominent regional power. They argue that following in the footsteps of Japan means women will be the primary caretakers of home and family.

When discussing gender and family norms around housework and childcare, JSA practitioners often refer interchangeably to "Asian tradition" or "Cambodian tradition." In doing so, they are sometimes referencing and, often, conflating the above dominant essentialist ideas about Cambodian culture that promote female chastity and assign women most of the household and childcare duties, alongside simplified Chinese Confucian norms (frequently generalized to all of Asia) that restrict women to their familial and household roles (Brickell 2011; Chen 2010; Rosenlee 2023).

Cambodian program managers list two reasons for reinforcing what they call Asian gendered beliefs. First, JSA managers are charged with befriending state officials who often hold similar beliefs about men and women's roles in the family. That means they find it appealing that JSA upholds these beliefs. Additionally, JSA's program managers express strong "traditional" beliefs about gender in Cambodian society in their own personal lives, which will be examined in more depth in the following chapter.

While they never discuss gender directly, JSA's Japanese staff did sometimes challenge managers' narratives about Asian gender norms. For instance, headquarters staff member Akari questions Boran—"How can women taking care of the home be the Asian way when all of your wives have jobs?" Japanese staff also notice the gendered dynamics at play, particularly in the division of labor during trainings. At a cooking training, Hanako laments that "not everyone is learning." She tries to engage men with the cooking activity. JSA's director, Junko, backs her up and informs her program managers that, in future, all health center staff should participate in the cooking training. But such interventions go largely ignored.

Also, at JSA, there is no discussion of reproductive health, family planning, menopause, or women's health outside of childbearing. At a training, one village volunteer asks JSA program managers if they plan to educate villagers on family planning at community health events. Junko responds that the staff will discuss the matter and get back to the volunteer. Over lunch, she tells me she worries about the cultural pressures on young Khmer women for early childbearing. Couples get married young, and they are pressured by their parents to have a child. Even if couples want to be smart and plan it out, their parents and grandparents can get mean and say she is not a good woman if she does not have a baby.

Later, Junko brings up this topic with her managers, couching it in terms of biomedical need. She explains that when doing the baseline survey, she met too many women who were pregnant at fifteen or sixteen years old. It is not healthy for the female body to bear children that young. She suggests, "we need to inform them that spacing births and not bearing children until twenty is necessary for good maternal health." But Sovann quickly jumps in to reject the idea that even a blanket statement such as this should be made at their trainings. He demands that birth spacing is a "difficult and political topic," outside the scope of JSA's project.

Khmer program managers swiftly rejected discussions of topics like reproductive choice because they are unwilling to take up any topic that might be deemed mildly political. Managers worry doing so might threaten their friendships with state officials. Japan's gender regime aims to upgrade women's place in society through better access to health knowledge and public services. However, JSA's project also implicitly assumes women will bear the burden of their own and their children's health. In practice, managers use the Asian imaginary to double down on these assumptions, even when they need to ignore Japanese managers to do so. They use JSA's project activities to advocate for the idea that traditional gender roles in the family are a key part of Asia's modern future.

HYBRIDIZING BIOMEDICAL AND "TRADITIONAL" MEDICINE

JSA staff also use a nuanced version of the Asian imaginary to hybridize project activities. As discussed above, for Japanese donors and practitioners, the modern Asian mother who uses "modern" medicine is juxtaposed to those who use "traditional" health practices. Instead of focusing on the role of the father or financial need as barriers to maternal health, which would require an intervention into gender or economic inequalities, Japanese INGOs focus on disparaging traditional medicine. The health report of another Japanese INGO implementing women's health activities in Cambodia makes this clear. It states:

> There was a woman in [location of Cambodian] village that did not trust the local health center at all. Instead, she entrusted her and her family's healthcare to a traditional birth attendant and a traditional healer in her village. She was comfortable asking her traditional birth attendant to assist her in delivery. She did not want to go to the health center, because she felt shy and was afraid of the health center staff. The health of her children was not very good, because she had limited knowledge of health and nutrition issues and hygiene conditions at her home were not very good. Then, a VHSG [public village volunteer] invited her to join in a health education activity organized by the VHSG, health center staff, and [INGO Name]. After this education activity, she understood the message and was not afraid to see health center staff. She takes her children to get vaccinated and for treatment when they are ill at the public health center. She has also cleaned her house, drinks only boiled water, and feeds her children more nutritious food. With these new habits, her family's health condition is much improved.

For Japanese donors and practitioners, doing away with "backwards" traditional medicine is a key goal of programming. Yet, resisting this, JSA staff and Cambodian public health staff work together to strategically shift the content of JSA's trainings when it comes to traditional health practices. Samnang tells me they do so because Japanese donor and manager directives do not give enough respect to the *yays* (grandmothers).

On my first day at JSA, Boran shows me the Cambodian Ministry of Health's policy on the "modern family." As Junko listens, he explains to me JSA is helping the ministry implement this policy here in Steung Treng province by "trying to change the low people's concept and help women become modern Asian mothers." He goes on to report that many village people believe in *kru khmi* (traditional healers), *chmop boran* (traditional birth assistants), and magic. If the healers say give your child sugar water, they will do it . . . but the modern mother, she gives only nutritious food to the child and she does not use the traditional practices.

Junko chimes in, saying this is particularly a problem if the *yay* (grandmother) has a lot of influence over the mother. Boran agrees, telling me that even if we teach the mother the right way, the yay might say "no, you must do it the way it has always been done, the way it was when I had children."

In conversations with Japanese staff, JSA's Cambodian staff members focus on the need to educate mothers into biomedical health practices. Sometimes they even join Junko in making disparaging remarks about traditional remedies.

However, when not in the presence of Japanese staff Sovann explains, it does not work just to tell villagers traditional practices are bad and their grandmothers are wrong. The elderly deserve more respect. Elder respect is upheld by practitioners as part of "Asian" tradition. It is also particularly significant in Cambodia where there are a limited number of elderly people due to the Khmer Rouge genocide and one's place in the social hierarchy is of great cultural importance (Jacobsen 2010).

To challenge Tokyo's discounting of traditional medicine, we see Khmer practitioners complicate their use of the Asian imaginary through inter-Asian referencing. Samnang uses examples from other Asian nations to challenge ideas coming from Japan. He asks me if I knew that in ancient times China and India were more advanced than Japan. Cambodian people have been using Chinese and Indian practices in the past, and those places still use traditional medicines now too. Here we can see the varying meanings of "tradition" and "modern" in the development imaginary. Managers draw on Asian similarity and esteem for Japan to reinforce so-called traditional Asian beliefs about gender. Yet, in the case of traditional medicine, Samnang brings in ancient China and India to challenge his Japanese bosses and the project's sole reliance on "modern" biomedical interventions.

In practice, JSA staff and government officials help public health workers promote a hybridization of biomedical and traditional maternal healthcare practices (Decoteau 2013). When asked by a village health volunteer about whether women should go to see the *kru khmi* (traditional healer), Samnang encourages her to tell women it is not a problem to see *kru khmi* as long as they see "the modern doctor" too. Traditional birth attendants also continue to play a role in maternal health in Cambodia, even more so for indigenous women. These attendants continue to advise women on what to eat, mix traditional medicines for expectant mothers, create ritual fires that warm a new mother's body, and assist with birth in some cases (Nikles 2008). Again, JSA managers and public health officials advocate for birth and prenatal care to take place in public health centers, but do not discourage women from seeking the services of the traditional birth attendant in tandem. Cooperation to hybridize project activities in this way is made possible by the close relationship between JSA staff and state officials detailed in chapter 2. Finally, I also often saw JSA staff themselves utilizing traditional cures, such as teas made by traditional healers or cupping.

Japanese aid envisions a strong public maternal health system in which Cambodian mothers can access public health services and increase their health knowledge. Nevertheless, the activities implemented to achieve this vision are modified by Cambodian practitioners using the Asian imaginary to reinforce "traditional" gender roles in the family as they hybridize "traditional" and "modern" medical practices.

U.S. Family Aid: "Women as Empowered Consumers"
WOMEN'S HEALTH AND THE U.S. GENDER REGIME

As discussed in chapter 2, U.S. donor and headquarter organizations prioritize upgrading private clinic and NGO provision of health services for women. The design of these projects is impacted by the U.S.'s gendered healthcare legacy, transnational feminist advocacy, and USAID's emphasis on a certain type of women's empowerment.

The design of U.S. women's health programs is informed by the U.S.'s history of private maternal healthcare and the assumption that public services should only be provided to the most marginalized. Unlike Japan, the U.S. healthcare system itself faces increasing challenges in providing adequate maternal healthcare. Among OECD nations, the U.S. has one of the highest maternal mortality rates. In 2000, the rate was 9.8 maternal deaths to every 100,000 live births. By 2014, it had more than doubled to 21.5 maternal deaths to every 100,000 live births. It has remained high in recent years, with the rate for 2022 continuing at approximately 22 maternal deaths to every 100,000 live births per year (Gunja et al. 2024; Nelson, Moniz, and Davis 2018). Maternal death in the U.S. is highly classed and racialized. In the U.S., black women are three to four times more likely to die in childbirth than white women, regardless of class background, with lower-class status only worsening outcomes further (Delbanco et al. 2019).

For American women, the default expectation is that prenatal, delivery, and reproductive healthcare are purchased in the private sector. As a result, upper- and middle-class women with private insurance typically seek care earlier and have better birth outcomes. Delivery costs are high in the U.S., at about 10,000 U.S. dollars for a vaginal birth without complications. As insurance typically covers only a percentage of this cost, women pay an average of 4,000 U.S. dollars per vaginal birth (Khazan 2020). Only for women in poverty do government programs subsidize care. In the 1980s, Congress expanded Medicaid to increase coverage of women in families below the federal poverty level with the goal of lowering infant and maternal mortality rates (Ellwood and Kenney 1995). Yet lower-class women continue to face barriers in access to adequate healthcare, particularly prenatal care. This legacy of a hybrid healthcare sector is exported to Cambodia through the U.S.'s emphasis on upgrading private and nonprofit services for women's health.

In terms of family planning, the U.S. Supreme Court gave married couples the right to use birth control in 1965. By 1972, after high levels of feminist mobilization, birth control was legalized for all citizens (Gibson 2015). Contraception is widely available and commonly used by American women. Reproductive control is understood to be essential for women to succeed in the workforce. Subsequently, U.S. donors and INGOs frequently implement family planning activities alongside maternal health programming.

In Washington, D.C., in contrast to Tokyo, discussions about gender equality are common. USAID's commitment to gender equality and women's empowerment is evident in interviewee rhetoric, USAID's prominent gender equality policy, the integration of gender-specific indicators into planning and evaluation, millions spent each year on gender-specific projects, and the fact the agency has gender experts on staff. USFA headquarters staff explain it is essential to make women's health programming "gender transformative" and "address the power relations between men and women." This emphasis on gender equality in the U.S. development sector is impacted by the legacy of transnational feminist organizing discussed in chapter 1.

Consequently, in the U.S. development sector, empowering women is an important goal, although it is also one that is currently facing backlash. Yet the empowerment embedded in the U.S. gender regime takes a specific form. In the U.S., empowerment "refers to individual accomplishment, achieved through education, economic self-sufficiency, and expanded consumer choices" (Radhakrishnan and Solari 2023: 41). This form of empowerment, and its prioritization of economic success, is baked into programs the U.S. exports to upgrade women's health abroad. For instance, a USAID report justifies its women's health activities with the following statement:

> Ensuring the survival and health of women is an imperative in its own right. But it is also a development priority because of the critical roles that women play in the nurture and education of their children as productive workers in their societies, as vibrant contributors of global economic growth, and as leaders in building democratic society (USAID 2014: 17).

Access to maternal health services and modern birth control methods are understood as essential to enable women's economic empowerment. USAID aims to empower women by giving them choices about what types of healthcare to consume, investing in NGO and private provision of maternal health and family planning activities.

Hybridization at U.S. Family Aid

USFA's project activities promote maternal health, reproductive health, newborn nutrition, water and sanitation, and malaria prevention: all activities USAID deems related to improving the health of women and children. It subcontracts to four local NGOs in rural areas to implement these activities and monitors their work each quarter. USFA staff also monitor a network of private clinics that provide maternal and reproductive health services to upgrade their quality of care.

USAID requires INGO implementers to conduct a gender analysis before project implementation can take place. To conduct the analysis, INGOs need to research gender norms and power relations between men and women in their project's context. Then the organization develops a plan of action for integrating gender throughout the project. In its plan, USFA commits to gender activities such as male integration into education about family planning, maternal health, and child nutrition to challenge unequal assumptions about who undertakes childcare. Additionally, USFA will also host a gender workshop for the staff of USFA's government partner (the Cambodian Center for Health Communication), include gender sensitive indicators in its monitoring and evaluation, and provide gender workshops for USFA staff and implementing partner organizations.

In consequence, staff at USFA do consider gendered power relations when addressing barriers women face in access to healthcare. In a meeting, the project team considers how to improve child and maternal nutrition; USFA's director, Ranny, chief of party, Dr. Belinda, and deputy director, Erin, discuss barriers to changing expectant mothers' eating habits, including financial need, geographical access, but also the support of husbands and in-laws. Ranny points out it is necessary to educate fathers as well as mothers on maternal health and nutrition. She says that in a previous project, fathers blocked women from seeing doctors because it was too expensive. She argues that in this case they need to design activities that follow the directives of donors and the "West" to promote gender equality. By educating men, women could be enabled by their spouses to become better healthcare consumers. This discussion, which addresses power relations in the home, is very different from conversations that take place at JSA.

Nevertheless, while the gender equality directives of the West can sometimes be seen as useful, staff at USFA also contend with the fact that the word "gender" itself is frequently understood to be a Western import in Cambodia. While transnational feminist groups have advanced women's economic and social position all over the world, there has been backlash against gender equality norms in many nations (Cupac and Tuncer-Ebeturk 2022). In Cambodia, this backlash often takes the form of accusing the West of pushing gender equality on the country. At a workshop on health behavior change, when the topic of gender arises, an older male staff member from the Cambodian Center for Health Communication responds in an annoyed tone. He argues that concern with gender is a foreign imposition. He states, "in our culture these days, woman is king, foreigners have pushed for women and men to be equal. There is no more difference between men and women because foreigners have pushed this on Cambodian culture." Such beliefs made it necessary to find creative ways of localizing discussions about gender equality. To do so, USFA staff begin "hybridizing" project activities by merging their understandings of "Western" and "Asian" gender norms in constructing the call for proposals to which subgrantees will apply.

USFA's communications manager, Srey-na, considers herself a feminist and contends that projects must challenge household gender norms to improve women's reproductive choices. In project activity design meetings, she argues that feminist beliefs are "not just for the West" but for everyone. In a meeting discussing family planning education activities, Dr. Belinda argues for the need for projects to empower women to make choices, although she does not think USFA needs to work with men. She expresses the belief that in "Asian families" men do not discuss such topics. Countering with a different vision of Asia, Srey-na responds carefully that "Asian families" value things like togetherness, cooperation, and community care, drawing on beliefs that the West is more individualistic than many Asian societies. Srey-na goes on to explain that if men are kept in the dark, they cannot support their wives in accessing medical birth control. However, Srey-na agrees that pragmatically, it may be difficult for implementing partner organizations to work with men. Therefore, in this meeting, they agree that requiring two to four events per year that include male partners is a good compromise.

Consequently, USFA displays an uneven, albeit pragmatic, commitment to its goal of challenging and transforming gender relations in Cambodia. In project design, USFA practitioners negotiate how to translate "Western" demands for gender equality into the Cambodian context, starting the process of hybridization. However, while USFA staff design and monitor health project activities, it is local NGO subgrantees that implement USFA's activities directly. To fully investigate the implementation of USFA's women's health activities, we need to examine how they are put into practice by staff at USFA's implementing partner, the Cambodian Development Society (CDS).[1]

Project Activities at the Cambodian Development Society

"We disperse health information, and we help young women and mothers with too many children buy the modern birth control."
    —REASMEY, CAMBODIAN DEVELOPMENT
    SOCIETY, HEALTH TEAM LEADER

The Cambodian Development Society (CDS) is contracted by USFA to provide education on family planning and maternal health in the rural villages of a province called Kampong Speu. Its target population is women of reproductive age, including young and recently married women, pregnant women, new mothers with children under two, mothers with more than four children, as well as women who employ "traditional" family planning methods, such as withdrawal. There is a clear emphasis on women's economic empowerment in CDS's work. As its contract states, CDS works on the "demand side" by encouraging women to visit, largely private, clinics and uptake modern birth control methods. CDS staff are training women to "advocate for their health" and "bring consumers into the healthcare market."[2] USFA's measurement plan flows from this directive. As we will see below, the requirements in this contract provide specific opportunities for and constraints on hybridization at CDS.

Due to the hybridization that begins at USFA, the contract between USFA and CDS includes aspirational gender rhetoric, noting the importance of empowering women through reproductive choice and the need to incorporate both men and women in educational activities. However, the contract only actually requires incorporating husbands and male community members into education events two to three times a year. As they put USFA's activities into practice, CDS staff hybridize the project further.

HYBRIDIZATION AT CAMBODIAN DEVELOPMENT SOCIETY

To observe project implementation, I travel around Kampong Speu province with Reasmey, the leader of CDS's health team. When she is not completing paperwork in CDS's office, Reasmey travels by moto (the Cambodian term for motorcycles and scooters) often for hours into the countryside, to observe the work of her health team. The health team is made up of twelve members: eleven women and one man. Each health team member oversees a target area of approximately three or four communes. Most team members live with their families in a village within their assigned target area. Health team staff members' foremost concerns are often solving the problems of rural poverty and helping their families make ends meet. This means debates around Asian and Western development models are less prominent at CDS than at USFA or JSA. Nevertheless, in discussions of gender and family, notions like "Asian families" and concerns about gender equality as a "Western import" still come up.

Health team members spend most of their time getting to know people in the villages in their assigned area and training small groups of women on maternal and reproductive health. In contrast to Japan Services Asia (JSA), where staff conduct some limited village mapping but mainly count on village health volunteers to gather information about target participants, CDS staff spend a lot of time building relationships with and gathering information about women of child-bearing age in their assigned villages.

One day, I went with Reasmey and her health team member, Sotarath, to complete a village mapping. When we arrive, Sotarath is in conversation with her uncle's friends, who live in the village. Based on informal discussions with villagers, Sotarath is drawing a map of the village. It documents access to water, rice farms, and nearby health centers. Each house in the village is drawn, with circles around the ones where women live that might need health education. We go together to visit another acquaintance of Sotarath. She fills us in on her neighbors, reporting to us women who have more than four children, those who recently had a baby, and those who travel to Phnom Penh for factory work.[3] After this, we go to visit the village chief. We lay out the map for him and he adds information to it, suggesting we visit one woman with five children who lives on the outskirts of the village.

In addition to mapping, health team members conduct health trainings. Trainings take place in women's homes and typically include no more than five family members, friends, and/or neighbors. To observe a training, I travel with Reasmey to a village approximately an hour and a half away from the provincial capital of Kampong Speu where CDS maintains its office. We wind slowly down bumpy dirt roads on her moto until we find the health team member, Chantou, waiting for us in a hammock at her aunt's home. Chantou takes us to observe her health training. We visit a mother, who cannot be more than fifty years old, and her two adult daughters. One daughter recently had a baby, and the other is pregnant. We sit in the shade beneath their wooden house on a bamboo platform. Two women from neighboring houses come over to listen as well, one with her own toddler and baby in tow. The babies sit looking at each other, getting jostled on their mother's laps. The mother of the house listens while weaving at her loom.

Reasmey and Chantou get to know the women a bit, inquiring about their families and holding their babies. Then Reasmey and Chantou get out their colorful pamphlets and pass them around. One boasts pictures of breastfeeding mothers and pregnant women at the health clinic. The other presents photos of different medical birth control methods. First, Chantou asks the women if they know how many times pregnant women and new mothers should visit the clinics for pre- and postnatal care, what pregnant women should eat, and how to breastfeed. The pregnant woman says it is hard to go to the clinic for a checkup because she needs to work. Chantou and Reasmey respond that they will help her talk to her husband and Chantou can drive her to the clinic. Reasmey exclaims, "I am sure your husband wants a healthy baby!"[4]

Next, Chantou asks the women if they know how soon after giving birth a woman can get pregnant, inquiring about the family planning methods they use. One mother says she has tried the pill while the rest of the women say they use traditional methods. After that answer, Reasmey launches enthusiastically into family planning education. She uses a "happy couples" booklet to discuss the need for family planning with husbands. Next, she explains each of the "modern" methods including the pill, the implant, the shot, condoms, and then takes extra time to promote the IUD.

I later discover the commitment to the IUD is due to organizational history. USFA strictly adheres to USAID's rules to promote all methods equally in project documents. But CDS had a previous project with a different donor in which the health team specifically encouraged IUD use. For this reason, it is the modern method with which health team members are the most familiar and encourage most fervently. After detailing the forms of contraception, the training conversation takes a serious tone as Reasmey and Chantou also tell the women that although a lot of people do not know it, abortion is also legal in Cambodia up to twelve weeks into a pregnancy.[5]

After Reasmey and Chantou's presentation, the participants look overwhelmed by all the information. They are also a bit nervous to be discussing the topic of family planning. One mother says her friend used the shot and it made her gain weight. Reasmey says this is possible, but that is why the nonhormonal IUD is better. The mother of the house chimes in, saying she tried the pill once, but it gave her hot flashes. Reasmey responds by explaining the hormones in the pill have been updated since that time. A pregnant participant says she has heard the IUD can make you infertile. Reasmey explains she has heard this too, but it is a myth, stating "sometimes we listen to hearsay, but it is better to listen to the midwives and doctors at the clinic."

Then, speaking quietly, the neighbor expresses her anxiety about the number of children she has. She tells Chantou she has three children. She does not think she can afford to have more. However, her husband does not want her to take birth control. Reasmey says this is another positive of the IUD. "There is a private aspect to it" and "no one but you and the provider have to know anything about it." Chantou supports this, explaining it will work for years, her husband will never know about it, and it can be removed at any time. After discussing their questions, Reasmey and Chantou quiz the women, asking them questions like "What is an IUD?" "How many prenatal visits to the clinic should pregnant women have?"

To conclude the visit, Chantou provides the women with referrals to nearby clinics. She promises to visit them again in a couple weeks. After the women disperse, Chantou speaks quietly to the neighbor, asking if she wants her to take her to the clinic to get an IUD when her husband is out of the house. While USFA aspires to include husbands and wives in discussions of family planning, in practice, health team members frequently aid women who want to utilize medical birth control without their husband's consent.

CDS's health team members are deeply aware of the needs of the communities they serve. In implementation, this project is very different from that of Japan Services Asia. It does very little to support public health services, as health staff engage with public health clinics only when no private clinic in USFA's network is nearby for beneficiaries to access. CDS's project also does not reinforce the power hierarchy of male state officials and public health workers. Of course, there are power dynamics between the female trainers and village participants. NGO workers are widely considered more educated and well paid than the average villager, commanding a certain level of respect. Still, it is not the same level of esteem given to male health experts, in front of whom village women feel obligated to act formally and limit their questions.

As we saw above, trainers and trainees have intimate conversations about difficult topics, and mothers are provided with choices about their reproductive health. After trainings are complete, health team members and beneficiaries chat about village happenings and who else might need this training. I hear several trainees express that they did not know about some of these contraception methods before. This is not just a transfer of government sanctioned maternal and child health information. Relationships are built between beneficiaries and staff, and health staff follow up with trainees to encourage health behavior change. Like JSA's beneficiaries, women receiving services from CDS are more interested in sussing out the place of individual health team members in village kinship hierarchies and what benefits they might provide rather than assessing CDS and the origins of its donors.

In addition to village mappings and small group trainings, CDS health staff need to conduct large community health workshops at least once per quarter. At health education workshops, pre- and postnatal care are described, health team members perform entertaining skits about breast-feeding, and all the types of medical birth control are discussed. After information is dispersed, participants play quiz games and those that can answer questions about maternal and reproductive health correctly are given prizes. At the community health education event I attend, there are about twenty women and one male in attendance. Reasmey tells me it is more difficult to get men to attend these events since men need to work away from the village during the day.

Yet, as required by USFA, CDS also holds "happy couple" events where model couples present their experience sharing decision-making about family planning and maternal health. Reasmey explains that happy couple events, which include both men and women, are held less frequently, maybe once or twice a year, and often later in the afternoon. "Happy couple" events are difficult because it is not so easy to find two couples willing to talk publicly about family planning, since it is seen as a "women's issue" and a "difficult topic" to discuss openly.

Reasmey tells me that to implement a larger number of happy couple events, USFA would need to provide more support so events could be held in the evening. She would need to pay health team members overtime for working at night and provide dinner to attendees. In practice, outside of required happy couple events, when men come in during trainings, they are often waved off by the trainers and trainees or run away as soon as they hear the issues being discussed.

In implementation, CDS staff further hybridize project activities. They maintain a firm focus on women, taking up incoming norms around gender equality selectively in response to community needs and staff perceptions. Reasmey informs me she believes women should have a choice in family planning; this is very important. She reports learning a lot about family planning choices from her interactions with Western INGOs. She encourages women to "take power on the issue of their health." But Reamsey is also aware that changing men's perspectives will "take a very long time" and women in the communities need to solve their family planning problems in the present. Despite rhetoric that men and women should be involved, in practice, the CDS health team strategically determines that with the resources USFA provides, it is more pragmatic to focus on supporting women's health choices.

Reasmey explains, "I don't know how you do it in your country," but birth control "is a woman's issue in Asian families." Reasmey tells me, in her own family, she feels the duty of birth control should fall to the wife "since she is the one who can get pregnant." She goes on to tell me condoms are only for the man to protect his family. She states, "sometimes the wife, we are tired, we cannot please him so he would go outside but he should also protect himself, not bring any disease into the family or let the community know of his actions. That is how to be a good husband."

Reasmey's statements about her personal life mirror the project's hybridization. She believes deeply in female choice and access to contraception but finds it more difficult to challenge men's power. Reasmey goes on to say she assumes in the West such topics are more open and that is why the donors want trainings that include men and women. Yet, even in the U.S., while discussions about birth control might be more open, in long-term relationships the responsibility for birth control also almost always falls to women (Littlejohn 2021).

Thus, unlike at JSA, staff at USFA and CDS do discuss women's empowerment through choice and address the "difficult" topic of reproductive health. However, CDS staff do not feel they have the time or resources needed to confront unequal gender household relations. Instead, they hybridize what they understand to be "Western" and "Asian" family norms, creating a project that focuses on women's choice, and doing what they feel is the most pragmatic to improve the lives of women in village communities. In this hybridization process, the intentions of donors in Washington, D.C., are hybridized or effectively "watered down" at both USFA and CDS. Nevertheless, women's knowledge about and access to medical birth control is improved through CDS's activities.

THE LIMITS OF HYBRIDIZATION AT
CAMBODIAN DEVELOPMENT SOCIETY

However, family planning and reproductive health projects can have dual consequences. These activities can give women access to medical birth control, providing them with control over their bodies. Fewer children can improve maternal health as well as work and education opportunities for mothers and children. But family planning projects can also re-create long-standing hierarchies in which poor women are assumed to be unworthy mothers whose reproductive capacity should be limited. At CDS, the legacies of both consequences exist side by side.

The previous section described the CDS health team's routine activities in project implementation. However, during quarterly evaluations, CDS staff find themselves particularly constrained by USFA's metrics. These time periods illustrate the limitations practitioners can face when employing the development imaginaries to modify project activities. USFA measures CDS's success in the number of women that staff convince to uptake medical birth control and the number of prenatal visits attended each quarter.

USAID has been a leader in promoting innovative measurement techniques in development since the 1960s. Agency leaders believe measurement and evaluation are an essential way to ascertain whether funds are being used effectively (Krause 2014). Additionally, in the recent past, USAID projects have been criticized for using the number of women trained as an indication of success but failing to provide evidence of behavior change. USAID pushes USFA to address this problem. CDS health team members are trained in health behavior change communication and provided with referral slips. Successful referrals are measured by the number of pre- and postnatal care visits and uptake of modern birth control. However, aid metrics can often have unintended consequences (Suh 2021).

When the time for quarterly evaluations draws near, staff feel pressure to meet their numbers so CDS can continue acquiring funding. This is not to say that many beneficiaries do not want to use medical birth control. Numerous training participants are happy to have the information and seek out medical birth control after getting a referral from CDS's health team. However, the number of women who do so is not always enough to meet the target quota. When this is the case, health team members find themselves in a position where they need to quickly convince more women to use medical birth control.

Team members use many methods to convince women to use modern birth control, such as allaying their fears or taking them to clinics themselves. On rare occasion, they also turn to misinformation. Chantou explains to traditional method users that withdrawal can be "dangerous" for their husband:

> You, who use the natural ways, do you know the consequences of the natural methods? You don't know? It impacts the health of your husband very much and he does not sleep so well . . . it is as if you are driving a motorbike that goes very fast, and we go down a slope at a very high speed and there is something that crosses the road and we brake abruptly . . . we fall, right? His nervous system will be excited, he will have psychological problems after this, it is like madness. He can't sleep and think a lot about it and some men will have weaknesses because he was not able to get things out [ejaculate]. His head and his body . . . this badly impacts his health. For the hormones in birth control, it impacts your health. But if you use natural ways, it impacts the health of your husband. Do you want that?

Such misinformation can serve to frighten women into using medical birth control to protect their partners.

Furthermore, about twice a year, CDS staff assist USFA quality assurance monitors. For this project, which receives funding from a different donor, USFA staff come to observe and evaluate midwives at private clinics to do a "quality check." Using their community connections, CDS staff bring in women from the surrounding community to obtain services. Typically, this is not so hard for pre- and postnatal visits, although there is some cajoling of women to pause their work or of male family members to provide the small fee for clinic visits. However, USFA medical experts also want to observe technical skills, such as IUD insertion. This means health team members must convince at least three to five women in the community to get an IUD on this day.

On the quality check day that I observed, I traveled around with Reasmey and Sotarath. First, we go to pick up a young woman with a toddler and a newborn. She immediately comes with us, thanking the women for coming to pick her up. She gets in the van after leaving the newborn with her parents and the toddler with her husband. But Reasmey informs me we still need at least two more women, but most women in the villages are "uneducated and afraid." We spend two hours traveling to five different family homes.

Reasmey and Sotarath desperately try to convince women to get IUDs. The first woman we visit lives in a rundown home. She weaves bathmats out of strips of cloth to sell at the local market. She sits on a small bamboo platform, while four young children and several chickens play in the dirt nearby. Reasmey tells her about the IUD calmly, but the woman says she does not want it. Reasmey tells her she can be empowered by the IUD and take it out at any time, but the woman does not want it. Sotarath asks the woman kindly, "please, sister" and explains to the woman why she does not need to be afraid of the insertion or side effects, but the woman still says she does not want it.

Then Reasmey speaks with more passion, urging her to look "at her situation," as she points to the decrepit house and her half-dressed children running around without shoes. Reasmey points out to the woman, "You are so poor; how can you want more children?" She persists in asking her how she can provide for her kids and "What kind of life they will have?" The woman looks embarrassed, but without meeting Reasmey's gaze, she shakes her head and again says that she does not want it. Then Reasmey tries to convince the woman's father, who is sitting nearby. He says to ask her husband, who is away. After this, Reasmey and Sotarath give up. We go to four other houses, where they try to convince women and/or male family members. Eventually, two other women consent to the IUD insertion and come with us to the clinic. At the clinic, USFA health experts watch as the clinic doctor consults with each woman and inserts an IUD.

Quality monitoring days like these greatly intensify the pressure for CDS staff to get women to use modern birth control. Nevertheless, this finding supports international development scholarship in other countries that documents how measurement and evaluation practices can undermine a donor's own aspirations to empower women with reproductive choices (Suh 2021). It also illustrates that some metrics can limit NGO practitioners' ability to hybridize donor gender regimes. While CDS practitioners critique the quantification of aid activities by the "West," strict metrics limit their capacity to modify the project using the development imaginaries.

Women's Health and Development Imaginaries

As they implement women's health programs, practitioners at JSA, USFA, and CDS encounter foreign interventions into their nation's gender order. Women's organizations in the Global South are no strangers to the critique that gender equality is a "Western" import. Critics frequently levy rhetoric about Westernization at some development activities, like gender equality, but not others, like technological assistance (Narayan 1997). Such critiques have become increasingly prominent with the global gender backlash movement. Yet, here we see that alongside questions about Western intervention, in Cambodia today, there are now debates around Asian development and its impact on gender relations. Cambodian practitioners utilize the development imaginaries in diverse ways to determine how to advance women's health in their nation. In doing so, they modify project activities and make claims about the place of women and men in Cambodian society.

At JSA, when it comes to gender, Khmer program managers and state officials combine the Japanese gender regime and notions of Asian tradition to reinforce gender norms that assume Cambodian mothers will continue to take on most of the household and childcare labor. At the same time, JSA staff and state officials draw on ideas about medical traditions in other East Asian nations to discount Japan's directive to disparage traditional medicine. In putting project activities into practice, JSA staff and state actors create a vision of modern Asia in which traditional medicine, and the wisdom of grandmothers and midwives, are respected.

In a two-step process, USFA and CDS staff hybridize notions of women's empowerment from the West and ideas about Asian families to make their work palatable to villagers. With USAID funding, USFA and CDS staff must contend with the rhetoric that their projects challenging gender inequalities are a "Western import." USFA and CDS staff hybridize project activities to focus on promoting women's choice in reproductive healthcare but ignore the goal of challenging gendered power relations in households. They do so by picking and choosing from schemas they consider to be from Asia and the West.

This chapter illustrated that skepticism around gender equality as "Western" is prominent in Cambodia. Nevertheless, many Cambodian practitioners still use learnings from Western donors' gender equality trainings couched in more palatable terms. For instance, USFA practitioner Srey-na argues Western donors are right that men need to learn about family planning for women to truly have full access to contraception. She frames teaching men about family planning in rhetoric that men would want to learn because Asian families care about community, harmony, and working together. Yet the individualized, economic-focused form of women's empowerment that is promoted by U.S. donors also enables CDS staff's pragmatic decision to hybridize project activities to focus mainly on female choice in contraceptive consumption, ignoring power relations between men and women.

Finally, we must note, the Asian development imaginary is often employed to endorse "traditional" gender relations that put the majority of childcare and household work on women in Cambodia, but not always. We saw this usage when JSA managers contend that the assumption women will be the main caretakers of children is the "Asian way." And we also saw Srey-na at USFA employ the Asian imaginary to recruit men to uphold values like community care for mothers and children. In the next three chapters, we will dive deeper into these varied usages of the development imaginaries by investigating each INGO workplace in more depth.

FOUR

Contested Work-Family Bargains

INGO Workplace Inequalities

On the way to a health department meeting, I am riding in the back of a Japan Services Asia (JSA) Suburban with a program assistant, Mony. I inquire if Mony wants to move up and be a manager one day. She tells me she's grateful to work here and help her family out for now, but that she will probably quit working at JSA once she has children. She feels it is best to focus on her children after giving birth, and she can still make some income selling vegetables from her garden. Then program manager Boran chimes in from the driver's seat. Invoking regional similarity, he tells me that I might not get it as an American, but, as JSA is a Japanese organization, it is understood that mothering takes priority over work for women in Cambodia. Boran is then chided by his Japanese director, Junko, who is riding in the passenger seat. She says Mony could become a manager if she learned to speak better English.

At U.S. Family Aid (USFA), it is a different story. One day, I am working on a PowerPoint with Sotheary, who is on the program staff at USFA. After we finish editing, she tells me her concerns about combining work and childcare. She explains that at USFA they expect both women and men to conduct fieldwork in rural areas frequently. Unfortunately, she faces a lot of tension from her parents and in-laws for taking these trips. Sotheary feels this is unfair, as her husband does not face this pressure when he travels for work. But, she explains, her in-laws and her own parents believe that in Asian families, mothers should be with their children, not traveling for work. She shrugs her shoulders, lamenting that she cannot be in two places at once. She says she wants to try to convince USFA to change its practices, giving respite from frequent travel to mothers of infants and young children. Yet, despite these family tensions, she tells me it is still her plan to move up and pursue a manager position at USFA.

In this and the following chapters, we take an in-depth look at JSA and USFA's work environments. The above two conversations introduce the different expectations of workers at JSA and USFA. In the past, researchers often assumed donor demands create homogenizing requirements for the "professionalization" of NGO workplaces. Professionalization pushes NGOs to prioritize employees with skills like balancing budgets, evaluating programming, writing grant proposals in English, and drafting reports for donors, instead of workers that have connections to grassroots constituencies (Alvarez 2009; Lemay-Herbert et al. 2020; Markowitz and Tice 2002). Due to professionalization, NGO workplaces are assumed to be similar around the world. While this push for professionalization does impact NGO work, recent studies show that different political cultures in donor countries encourage distinct organizational policies in foreign aid agencies and INGOs (e.g., Dietrich 2021; Stroup 2012; Wilks 2019). I expand these findings to illustrate that donor differences set the stage for distinctive work environments, which are further modified by local practitioners.

The current chapter illustrates that development takes place in deeply gendered workplaces. Workplaces are not gender neutral; instead, gendered assumptions are infused into hiring practices, organizational policies, manager beliefs, and worker contracts (Acker 1990). The question of how women should combine work and motherhood, a key aspect in the debate about women's ideal place in advanced societies, is one that workplaces play a role in solving (Hays 1998). Consequently, donor gender regimes foster different expectations about the ways men and women will combine work and family responsibilities.

At JSA, Japan's gender regime draws on the history of a strong developmental state that prioritizes lifetime employment for men and economic growth. In Japan, this model historically meant women were relegated to temporary jobs (Shire and Nemoto 2020; Walby 2020). Contrastingly, at USFA, the donor gender regime emphasizes the integration of women and men "equally" into a liberal market economy, despite the demands of motherhood and childcare (Radhakrishnan and Solari 2023). In response, INGO staff employ schemas from the development imaginaries to articulate new beliefs about the correct way of combining work and family in Cambodia, modifying INGO workplace practices in the process. However, before analyzing the gendered work expectations at each INGO, I look more broadly at the context of gender, family, and work in Cambodia.

Gender and Work in Cambodia

For most of Cambodian history, women and men have both worked (Jacobsen 2008). Since the 1990s, in its pursuit of capitalist growth, the Cambodian government further encouraged women to enter the formal workforce to speed economic development (Brickell 2011). The Cambodian Labor Law of 1997 dictates "Khmer citizens of either sex" should receive equal pay, the right to unionize, and the right to strike. Due to this history and current policy framework, Cambodia has the highest female labor force participation rate in East Asia and the Pacific region, with 80 percent of women working in the country in comparison to 90 percent of men (Gavalyugova and Cunningham 2020).

Nevertheless, gendered work inequalities remain a problem in Cambodia. The Cambodian Labor Law of 1997 also dictates that women should not lose their jobs due to pregnancy and that women working for formal organizations are entitled to ninety days of maternity leave, during which they will receive at least half their wages (Council for the Development of Cambodia 2024). However, it's estimated that approximately 88 percent of Cambodians work in the informal labor market, meaning paid maternity leave can only be taken by a privileged few (ILO 2019). Additionally, despite legal rhetoric that men and women should receive equal pay, Cambodia has a wage gap with men earning more than women (Gavalyugova and Cunningham 2020). This is due to several factors. First, despite improvements in recent generations, on average Cambodia's labor force continues to have a low level of education, with women being at a particular disadvantage.

Strong cultural norms expect men to be breadwinners and women to bear the majority of the burden in caring for the home and children. Cambodian men are expected to protect and provide for their families. Wealth is a sign of a successful and marriageable man (Jacobsen 2011). Women are more likely than men to engage in informal microbusinesses, like selling their craft from home or subsistence farming. The likelihood of a woman working in nonwage, at-home employment increases after her first child is born (Gavalyugova and Cunningham 2020). Finally, there are few women in management and leadership positions in the economic and political spheres (UN 2020).

Nevertheless, within this long history of women's labor force participation, many Cambodians argue that a "good" woman earns a living for her family (Brickell 2011). However, this only goes so far—modern women are expected to have "respectable" jobs that require daytime labor such as office work or retail. But many women in the service sector, like servers at restaurants or bars, must work during nondaytime hours. When women do this kind of work in Cambodia it is stigmatized, often being equated with sex work, whether workers engage in that or not (Jacobsen 2008). Stigmatized jobs are more likely to employ lower-class and migrant women. Limited job opportunities in rural areas mean that women frequently must migrate to urban areas to engage in low-paid or precarious labor such as garment work, service work, or sex work (Derks 2008).

In this context, JSA and USFA practitioners work in "respectable" office jobs. Nevertheless, they must negotiate these dominant cultural beliefs around the appropriate combination of work and family. Here again, practitioners draw on notions of "traditional" and "modern" gendered beliefs alongside competing development imaginaries to reinforce, contest, and modify gendered work expectations.

The Donor Gender Regime and Work at Japan Services Asia

Three aspects of Japan's donor gender regime (discussed in chaps. 2 and 3) contribute to JSA's workplace practices: the implicit assumption that men are primary breadwinners and women are caretakers, the limited explicit discussion of gender inequalities, and the presumption that the state will be the primary agent of development.

First, the Japanese labor market's legacy influences its donor organizations and INGOs. Throughout the 1970s, Japan provided tax incentives for families with stay-at-home wives and the availability of nonfamily child or elder care was very limited, producing a familial welfare state (Takegawa 2009). Traditionally, in this model there was a strong gendered division of labor (Boling 2015; Ochiai 2014). Firms provided male breadwinners with long-term jobs. In contrast, women were often relegated to temporary or lower-paying employment, as it was assumed their income was supplemental to a male partner's or they would quit the job after childbirth (Ogasawara 1998; Peng 2012). However, with low fertility rates, by the 1980s, Japan began to pass laws to promote work-family balance to encourage female labor force participation alongside childbearing. The Japanese government passed the Equal Employment Opportunity Act in 1985, and during the 1990s expanded the provision of childcare and parental leave (Estevez-Abe 2014; My 2013; Peng 2012). Such policies have played an important role in changing the gendered labor market in Japan.

Nevertheless, the male breadwinner model is still embedded in workplace culture in Japan. Climbing the corporate ladder comes with an expectation to work incredibly long hours (Neomoto 2012). In 2016, approximately 75 percent of Japanese women aged twenty-five to fifty-four worked full time, up from 65 percent in 2000. However, approximately 33 percent held part-time jobs and less than 10 percent had managerial positions (comparatively 30 percent of women hold managerial positions in the U.S.) (Shambaugh, Nunn, and Portman 2017). As we will see below, JSA's hiring practices echo the Japanese "familial" welfare state and its inherent assumptions about men's and women's roles in the workforce (Ochiai 2014).

Second, as discussed in chapter 3, in stark contrast to INGOs funded by the U.S., there are no workshops on gender equality for staff, or any discussion of gender norms or inequalities in Cambodian society. When asked about gender, Japanese donor and INGO interviewees in Tokyo explain that Japan does "not intervene in Cambodian culture." Others tell me that being outspoken about gender is not the Japanese way. This is in line with research that terms feminism in Japan as a "quiet" or "silent" revolution in which women do not directly critique gendered inequalities. Instead, to move up in their careers, women choose silent tactics of resistance like simply refusing to get married or have children, working for foreign firms with different gender expectations, and/or choosing to leave Japan all together (Mandach and Blind 2021; Miller 2003). Nevertheless, JSA's lack of engagement with direct gender equality rhetoric means practitioners have limited tools to discuss gender in the workplace.

Third, Japan's donor preferences for supporting the developmental state influence JSA's hiring practices. Japanese staff argue it is necessary to hire male managers to be successful in supporting the Cambodian state. Being male makes it easier for managers to form relationships with public health officials, who are typically also men.

JSA'S HIRING PRACTICES

Working in this donor gender regime, the first level of JSA staff are the program managers, Chakra, Sovann, Samnang, the head manager, Boran, and the accountant, Atith. Managers are all male and between approximately thirty-five and fifty-five years old. Some program managers have expertise in the healthcare field. Two program managers, Samnang and Sovann, were hired because they had training in public health and nursing. The head manager, Boran, was given the opportunity to train to become a doctor during his tenure at JSA. To focus on building relationships with Steung Treng officials, staff spend much of their time in JSA's provincial office (with upper-level staff working in JSA's Phnom Penh office for only a few days each month). Program managers all speak English at an intermediate level and live in Phnom Penh. We travel to Steung Treng by van together each week.

The second level of program staff at JSA are program assistants. Program assistants all live in and are from Steung Treng province because it is their job to be community liaisons and provide knowledge of the local area to program managers. Program assistants are largely female and paid significantly less than managers. Assistants help managers and public health officials interact with village mothers and children at community health events. They also gather relevant knowledge about village community members and make follow-up visits to mothers. All program assistants are hired soon after the competition of high school or college (without medical training). One exception, a program assistant named Chea, completed her midwifery training just before beginning work at JSA. All program assistants speak limited English and struggle to communicate in staff meetings conducted in English. With these hiring practices, JSA creates a gendered hierarchy within its own organization of "expert" managers with biomedical knowledge and "indigenous" assistants with community knowledge (Akpan 2011).

Explaining JSA's hiring practices to me, Samnang states program assistants "don't stay so long." In the four months I spent at JSA, two program assistants left the organization. One quit because she found a better-paying job at a microfinance institution and the other left after getting married. Turnover in INGOs is not uncommon, and the vast majority of INGOs with funding from the U.S., Europe, and Australia experience high staff turnover. However, at JSA, turnover is largely an issue when it comes to program assistants. While moving up to the position of manager is theoretically possible, JSA staff report that often assistants stay in the position only temporarily, leaving when they find a better job opportunity, need to help on their family's farm, get married, or have a child.

In contrast, the program managers, Chakra, Atith, Boran, Sovann, and Samnang, have been working for JSA for ten, fifteen, eleven, nine, and six years, respectively. In part, this is because, unlike U.S. INGOs, which hire new staff when receiving a four-to-five-year grant and often lay off some project staff when the grant is complete, JSA is committed to projects for approximately ten years. Japanese staff find alternative sources of funding to continue the same work when one grant ends. Additionally, two years ago JSA moved from Kampong Speu province to its current project site, Steung Treng, to implement maternal and newborn health activities in a new area. When it made this move, JSA kept its program managers on while hiring new program assistants familiar with the new province. JSA also has two full-time Japanese staff members, the director, Junko, and her assistant, Hanako. Japanese staff from headquarters in Tokyo fly in at least twice a year and stay for several weeks.[1]

These hiring practices mean JSA follows the Japanese gender regime of promoting long tenure for upper-level male staff with a short-term female workforce. The hierarchical division of labor between program managers and assistants is firmly policed by managers. Program assistants must refer to managers as *lou kru*, or teacher, a respectful title in Cambodia. Program managers are highly directive of assistants' daily tasks, and managers spend substantial time training assistants to do new tasks correctly, such as writing receipts. Managers also let assistants know it is their job to deal with "women's problems" like building relationships with mothers and newborn babies during the village trainings.

Finally, in stark contrast to USFA, no Khmer staff member at JSA has experience in international development or working for an NGO before coming to work at JSA. Instead, further illustrating JSA's commitment to state-led development, four of JSA's staff have family members who work for the Cambodian government. For instance, program manager Samnang's father worked for the Ministry of Education for many years and is now an advisor to the king of Cambodia.

In another example, Junko explains why she hired one program assistant, Mony, over more qualified candidates. Compared to candidates with a college degree or advanced English skills, Mony has only a high school education and previous experience working as a maid. But Junko informs me that Mony's husband works at a public health clinic, and she believes up-grading Mony's health knowledge will transfer to her husband. In contrast to many donors and INGOs from the U.S., Europe, and Australia, JSA does not prioritize hiring workers with development skill sets like report or grant writing, instead favoring workers with connections to the state and healthcare backgrounds. Below, I investigate how JSA's practitioners modify these gendered workplace practices through the use of development imaginaries in their everyday work lives.

JSA's Workplace Inequalities: Men as Primary Earners

Encountering the donor gender regime and hiring practices at JSA, em-ployees have different responses. Cambodian managers employ the Asian imaginary to reinforce a workplace where men are the primary earners. But this does not go without contestation as Japanese staff and some program assistants try to resist and modify the gendered assumptions embedded in JSA's hiring practices.

CAMBODIAN MANAGERS REINFORCE "TRADITIONAL" GENDER NORMS

Cambodian managers interpret JSA's work environment through the Asian imaginary to reinforce patriarchal gender norms in work and family in Cambodia. JSA's program managers and some assistants espouse what they interchangeably refer to as "traditional Cambodian" or "traditional Asian" beliefs about gender and family life, expecting women to take on the ma-jority of childcare and household duties and men to earn the higher salary. Program managers express two reasons for traditional beliefs. First, it is strategic, allowing them to form better relationships with influential, male government officials that typically express similar beliefs. Second, for man-agers and some assistants, many "traditional" beliefs about the roles of men and women in society are true to their personal beliefs.

JSA program managers often expressed the belief that while both gen-ders should work, the man's job is "primary." Over steaming bowls of kuy teav (a Cambodian noodle soup similar to pho), Samnang and I discuss his upcoming nuptials. He explains to me his fiancée will not be a "modern wife" like me—traveling out to Steung Treng each week with four male program managers and their driver makes me "modern" in his eyes (in Cambodia, women do not traditionally travel unaccompanied by a family member). Samnang says his fiancée will be a "good Asian wife" who takes care of the house, the kids, and cooks his favorite meals like *samlaw koko* (a very tasty Cambodian vegetable soup) while he travels for work.

However, when I ask about her job, he laughs "of course, she will always work." His fiancée must also keep her job at a bank in Phnom Penh for "family stability." Samnang argues Japan and Cambodia share the similar perspective that women's main role is caring for the family, even though Cambodian women do not yet have the "privilege" of staying home as often as Japanese women do. Thus, the "Asian" imaginary is used flexibly by managers to adapt Japan's gender regime to the Cambodian reality in which wives frequently must work.

Boran and Sovann are both married and maintain similar perspectives when asked about their families. Sovann says he misses his children, but it is his wife's job to care for them and work nearby their home in Phnom Penh. Boran explains that these hiring practices are part of why he wants to work for an Asian organization instead of a Western one. He knows that Western INGOs explicitly try to challenge social norms around gender and family, practices he sees as hindering the future of Cambodia.

Similarly, when I inquire about their future plans, most female program assistants express the desire to get married as their foremost concern. But Sopheap and Chea report they want to further their careers first. However, Sopheap explains to me that, unfortunately, the managers are right and, particularly in the rural area where she lives, there is so much pressure for young women to get married. A good marriage and grandchildren are how a woman makes her parents very proud.

When JSA's donor gender regime meets Cambodian reality, Cambodian managers utilize the Asian imaginary to reinforce JSA's hiring practices and division of labor through beliefs about the responsibilities of women as the main caretakers in families. However, other staff at JSA try to resist the way managers reinforce Japan's gender regime.

JAPANESE STAFF AND PROGRAM ASSISTANTS' RESISTANCE

The reinforcement of traditional gender roles using the Asian development imaginary is resisted by Japanese staff and several program assistants at JSA. Despite unwillingness to directly discuss gender inequalities, JSA's Japanese staff, Junko and Hanako, do try to undermine these ideas in several ways. It may seem surprising at first that it was Japanese staff who attempted to modify the workplace assumptions inherent in the donor gender regime, but, as the below findings demonstrate, we cannot conflate the ideologies of development donors with the workers sent to implement them.

The first way Japanese staff challenge JSA's workplace inequalities is in their own lifestyles and the choice to have opted out of the gendered expectations of their own country. Now in her late fifties, Junko left Japan in the late 1980s to study to be a nurse in Hawaii. When Japanese public interest in Cambodia grew in the early 1990s, Junko decided to go to Cambodia to work in a hospital. Junko now lives in Cambodia permanently, is married to an American NGO director, and speaks Khmer. She describes Japan fondly, particularly in terms of the food and landscape, but she also explains that Japanese people are "very polite," "they have certain expectations," and it is easier for her to live in Cambodia without these expectations. Leaving Japan in the 1980s, Junko bucked the gendered traditions of her time with the decision to live and work internationally, as well as to not have biological children.

Hanako recently got her master's degree in Europe and then moved to work for JSA in Cambodia. She is also long-distance dating a Northern European man and returns to Japan infrequently. One day at JSA, during break time at a training, I ask Sovann about his family. As he explains that it is the wife's job to stay near the home and care for the family in Asia, Hanako quickly snaps back, "Well, why am I here?" By leaving Japan to work in Cambodia, Junko and Hanako use their own life experiences to challenge the narrative of "traditional Asian" women that program managers espouse.

Junko and Hanako are also aware of and complain about the gendered work inequalities in their organization, particularly in the relations between program managers and assistants. Junko describes this as a "hierarchy problem," instead of directly discussing gendered workplace inequalities. When she arrived at JSA three years ago, the "hierarchical" hiring practices were already well established. To combat her so-called hierarchy problem, during my time at JSA, Junko decided to hire two male program assistants and a female assistant with medical expertise, Chea (a midwife). Over lunch, she lets me know she thinks this will change the power dynamics in her workplace.

Junko also takes a special interest in female assistants that want to upgrade their technical skills and further their careers. She requests that Sovann teach Sopheap to drive the car when she expresses interest in it. She also asks me to tutor Sopheap and Mony in English to build their skills so it would be possible for them to become managers. Mony is largely disinterested in our English lessons, but Sopheap works hard to improve her language skills. One day, as we are riding in the backseat of the car together, Sopheap tells me quietly that she hopes "women can move up to be managers at JSA . . . not only in the American organizations," using the comparison to the West to question the masculinized hierarchy managers reinforce in the organization.

Unsurprisingly, at JSA, workplace tension arises from the fact that the program managers are all men who express so-called traditional gendered beliefs, and yet they work in an organization where the lead Japanese staff members, Junko and Hanako, are women. When Japanese staff try to up-grade the skills of Cambodian managers, there is frequently resistance. For instance, Hanako helps program managers fill out budgeting forms correctly, checking their work carefully. Junko also offers advice to managers on how to manage assistants. Boran, Sovann, Atith, and Samnang do not openly contradict Junko or Hanako, but they resist in passive ways.

One day, a visiting JSA staff member from Tokyo, who is female and about thirty years old, checks Boran's report and makes numerous corrections in front of the whole staff. After she walks away, Samnang asks Boran (in English to ensure my understanding), "You're the head manager, why do you need to take orders from a little girl?" In another example, Junko downloads a typing program and insists Boran use it to learn to type faster in English. He agrees but when she goes back to her office, the managers look at one another in annoyance and he does not use the program.

Boran, Atith, Samnang, and Sovann rationalize working for women by explaining to state officials, program assistants, and one another that their "real boss" is in Japan. The real boss they refer to is a Japanese man, Dr. Nagao. Dr. Nagao is one of the founding members of JSA and comes to visit the Cambodian office on occasion to assist in project implementation and evaluation. The program managers have all met Dr. Nagao and they praise him as a mentor who is respectful, caring, intelligent, and "a kind Asian man." Samnang directly compares his leadership style to Junko's: "She is authoritarian and communist [a particular insult in Cambodia as it harks back to the violent, communist Khmer Rouge regime], and he is gentle." This mental gymnastics in which their "real boss" is Dr. Nagao allows them to imagine themselves within a hierarchy with a man at the top.

In response to Junko's new hires of two male program assistants and a midwife to solve JSA's "hierarchy" problem, program managers did substantial work to reestablish the workplace hierarchy. Compared to the original female assistants who are high school graduates, managers rank the new male program assistants and Chea, who all have college degrees, as higher than the original assistants but lower than themselves. For instance, Sovann writes every staff member's name and position in hierarchical order on the board. He then explains the roles of managers and assistants, reinforcing the chain of command to the newcomers. Assistants are harshly policed for disregarding the communication flow required by this hierarchy, such as asking Junko a question without checking with a manager first.

Managers use not just gender but also sexuality to engage in this organizational boundary work that places them at the top of the hierarchy (Lamont and Molnar 2002). Boran goes so far as to call the new male program assistants "fruity," disparaging their sexuality and masculinity to reestablish workplace hierarchy. One male program assistant did identify as queer, but the other did not. Managers see that Junko is attempting to disrupt the organization's order with her new hires, and they use the Asian imaginary to interpret resistance to the gender order as dangerous to Khmer culture.

Junko, Hanako, and the program assistants are largely not successful in changing JSA's organizational practices, as JSA's workplace inequalities are strictly reinforced by Cambodian managers. However, they do illustrate that we cannot assume that expatriate staff are always in alignment with their donor's intentions. Nevertheless, two years after I left JSA, I checked in with some staff members on a follow-up trip to Cambodia. Sopheap told me she felt pressured by her family and Cambodian managers to quit her job at JSA after she gave birth to her son. The one straight male program assistant Junko hired in my time there was the only assistant to move up into a manager role.

JSA's hiring practices, which reflect the gender regime of Japan and are meant to serve the organizational mission to cooperate with state officials, are used by Cambodian managers to reinforce particular work and family relations in Cambodia. Cambodian managers are largely successful in resisting Japanese managers' and program assistants' challenges to JSA's gendered hierarchy in workplace interactions.

The U.S. Donor Gender Regime and Work at U.S. Family Aid

The donor gender regime in which U.S. Family Aid (USFA) is embedded creates very different workplace inequalities. USFA workplace inequalities are influenced by the legacy of the U.S. emphasis on market-based solutions, including women's economic empowerment, as well as USAID policies that require workers be educated about gender inequalities.

First, the U.S. has a residual welfare state, which provides limited social services to push citizens under the age of sixty into the market. The main welfare programs provided in the U.S. include Social Security, which provides citizens with limited retirement benefits after the age of sixty-two, and Temporary Assistance to Needy Families (TANF). TANF provides only limited, short-term assistance to the poorest families, pushing mothers (who make up over 80 percent of recipients) into the labor market (Morash 2024; U.S. Department of Health and Human Services 2012).

Consequently, American mothers have high rates of labor force participation, often due to the economic need of their families (Vandenberg-Daves 2014). Fifty-seven percent of American women are in the labor force. In 2019, among married couples, 48.8 percent are in families in which both spouses work and only in 19 percent of American families does only the husband work (U.S. Bureau of Labor Statistics 2019). Single mothers are even more likely to be in the workforce, at a rate of about 77 percent (Livingston 2018; U.S. Bureau of Labor Statistics 2019).

Paid parental leave is not a legal entitlement in the U.S. The only federal policy available for leave is the Family Medical Leave Act (FMLA). Passed in 1993, the act allows employees to take 12 weeks of unpaid leave to care for a family member, new child, or recover from a serious illness. Childcare in the U.S. is also largely privatized, meaning access to care and the quality of that care are dependent on ability to pay (Estevez-Abe 2014). Contributing to the lack of work-family policies, historically American feminists have centered equal female labor force participation and individual equality. For example, the U.S. is a leader in passing sexual harassment policies that support women as productive workers (Zippel 2006). Yet, it is the least generous of industrialized, wealthy nations in terms of work-family policies (Arellano 2015). Privileging market solutions and individual responsibility, the U.S. promotes a model of women's empowerment that prioritizes employment and pays little attention to the difficulties women face balancing work and family (Cummins and Blum 2015; Radhakrishnan and Solari 2023).

Following the U.S.'s own limited family policies, the donor gender regime in which USFA is embedded promotes hiring practices that assume male and female workers are equal, while ignoring the demands women may be more likely to face as caregivers. INGO practitioners and donors in Washington, D.C., place a high emphasis on hiring women practitioners. One USFA staff member in Washington, D.C., states, "all our INGO country offices need to be trying to hire 50/50 male-female." Headquarters staff explain they see INGOs as a great space to advance women's careers.

USAID also requires that INGO grantees work to address gender inequalities in both project implementation and workplace practices. When I ask how gender inequality is addressed by USFA globally, a headquarters interviewee explains:

> I feel very, very strongly that gender equity is an issue that should shift [what they are doing] every department at USFA. It's not a separate category of work. It's the way we should be doing our work, right, which is to understand—we work in health. There's no part of health that isn't affected by gender roles. So, in every program that we run, we should be thinking about the way that gender inequities in gender roles are shaping people's access to and uptake of health services. We should be trying to—the minimum is to make sure we're not doing harm by reinforcing gender norms that are destructive, right? . . . We're trying to open access for women. We're also trying to ensure that we're trying to challenge norms that keep men from using health services or [as not] seeing themselves as people who deserve or need health services or even [receiving services] as a weakness. We're trying to make sure that other gender identities and sexual identities are being included and thought about and that we're doing that in a way that's also kind of rational and proportional to the overall health problem that we're trying to solve. We need to be addressing these things in our workplaces and in our programming. So that means addressing sexual harassment in the workplace and including all gender and sexual identities there as well. That's the goal.

As we can see, headquarters staff have high ambitions for the way gender should be integrated into all aspects of USFA's work, including not just health interventions but also workplace policies. This means USFA staff have professional development workshops directly discussing gender in the workplace; they examine topics like sexual harassment or the importance of women's representation in management positions. Staff also have "gender sensitivity" trainings in which they learn how to integrate topics like gender equality, women's empowerment, or LGBTQ+ issues into INGO project activities. These opportunities mean USFA's Cambodia staff use language that directly addresses gender inequalities to critique the inherent problems with the way work and family are combined at USFA.

USFA HIRING PRACTICES

Khmer staff at USFA are approximately fifty-fifty male-female, with both men and women filling managerial roles. USFA hires staff that have experience working in other NGOs, private research firms that specialize in international development, bilateral aid agencies, and multilateral agencies, like the United Nations or the Asia Development Bank. USFA's director, Ranny, informs me that in her hiring process she values credentials and development experience, and that she tries to hire women when possible. USFA's hiring practices align with studies that show most NGOs are more likely to hire middle-class, educated, and urban workers (Lemay-Herbert et al. 2020).

All Khmer staff on the USAID project team are over twenty-five years old. The majority are married with children, except for two women who are still single and living with their family of origin. USFA's fifteen full-time staff members on the USAID project are organized into two teams: programming, and monitoring and evaluation. There is also a staff member charged with the budget, a research coordinator that bills part of her time to the project, a communications officer, and the chief of party. Finally, the chief of party answers to USFA's director, Ranny, and deputy director, Erin, who also spend 30 to 60 percent of their time on the USAID health project. Of the staff, the chief of party, Dr. Belinda, and deputy director, Erin, are foreign-born (Belinda is from the Philippines and Erin is American), while all other staff are Khmer. Headquarters staff make frequent visits to assist with different aspects of the project.

The work environment at USFA is cordial and professionalized. All meetings are conducted in English and all staff are fluent. USFA employees are often quite busy, rushing to complete the next activity on their list. This environment is spurred on by Erin, the American deputy director, who demands a fast-paced work environment. She believes that Cambodians will "mosey" if allowed, taking two-hour lunch breaks and naps (it is tradition in Cambodia to nap after lunch). Erin often enters meetings to speed up conversations or visits staff in their cubicles to ask when their work product will be complete.

At USFA, hierarchy matters, but to a much a lesser degree than at JSA.

There is great respect given to USFA's female director, "Madam" Ranny. Program and evaluation team members are given direction on their daily or weekly tasks from their team directors. Otherwise, staff refer to one another as *bong* (literally translated as "sibling"), a sign of friendship and equality in Cambodia. In the next section, I investigate how workers make sense of the rhetoric about the importance of workplace gender equality coming from USAID alongside the gendered work inequalities they face at USFA.

USFA Workplace Inequalities: The Grandparent Dilemma

At USFA, encountering the U.S. gender regime and its resulting hiring practices, Cambodian workers embrace some gendered work policies they associate with the West. Yet, at the same time, they utilize schemas from the Asian imaginary to resist what they see as problems with the Western work model. In doing so, Khmer staff advocate for a hybrid workplace.

Several male workers report that exposure to ideas challenging gendered household norms at USFA made them realize the importance of "not putting it all on women." For instance, project staff member Arun says he knows from being exposed to the "Western way" at USFA that it is "his duty" to also engage in housework and care for his children anytime he can. He explains that in taking some of his wife's load, she has been happier, and their relationship has improved. However, Arun clarifies that he does not do too much since he wants his wife to feel like a "good mother." He tells me that for women in Cambodia, caring for one's children well is a point of pride.

This desire to combine Western and Asian ideas about gender roles at work and in the family as Arun does is prominent at USFA. But it becomes more difficult when female workers try to combine the idea that men and women should be equal in the workforce with prominent cultural beliefs about a good wife and mother in Cambodia. Like Sotheary at the beginning of the chapter, female practitioners struggle to combine a successful professional life and what they call Asian family expectations around household labor and childcare. Often, this leads them to rely on extended families for childcare needs, particularly grandparents (Shu and Chen 2023).

A program staff member, Srey-na, and her husband both work in Phnom Penh. But they have two young children, and their jobs do not pay enough to purchase childcare, which is limited in Cambodia and largely only affordable for expatriates or wealthy Cambodian political and/or business-owning families. So, Srey-na and her husband leave their children with her husband's parents in a rural town in Takeo province each week, traveling upwards of three hours to see them, and only on weekends. Srey-na's in-laws make her, but not her husband, feel guilty for not being with her kids every day.

Due to this guilt, two years ago, Srey-na took a job at a small NGO in Takeo. However, she found this job "boring, repetitive, and unprofessional," compared to fast-paced INGO work in Phnom Penh. Srey-na reports she decided to find another job back in Phnom Penh: "I like the work, I like the clothes, I like the lifestyle here. . . . I just couldn't stay out there. . . . I felt like I wasn't successful in my career anymore." In coming back to Phnom Penh, she continues to face tension from her in-laws.

Monitoring and evaluation specialist Chantrea also says it is difficult to be a good mother, a good wife, and a good development professional. She recently had a baby, and daycare is too expensive for her and her husband to afford. Her parents care for her baby while she works each day, but they live on the outskirts of Phnom Penh on the complete opposite side of town from Chantrea and her husband's home (largely only expatriates, wealthy businesspeople, longtime residents, and political families can afford to live centrally in Phnom Penh). To solve this problem, Chantrea and her new baby stay with her parents during the week while her husband and son stay at their house on the other side of Phnom Penh. She only sees her immediate family on the weekends.

About a month into my observation at USFA, Chantrea is asked to travel for three weeks of fieldwork to conduct monitoring and evaluation research in the provinces. Chantrea tries to express to her manager, Panh, that this is a difficult time for her to make a field visit, but Panh informs her such visits were in her job description. Yet the need to travel adds stress on top of her already trying childcare arrangements. To make the trip, she will need to stop breastfeeding early, although she has been doing so for only eight months, and she had planned to breastfeed for a year.

Additionally, she is stressed by her family's concerns about her travel for work. This is because, a few years ago when Chantrea traveled to the field with a different INGO, she was in a serious car accident; the car Chantrea was riding in flipped, the driver was killed, and Chantrea's arm was crushed. She had to travel to Thailand for surgery and mobility in her right arm is permanently impaired. Chantrea worries that frequent travel by car to the field is not safe, as many NGO workers experience car accidents.

She explains that in Cambodia a "good Khmer woman" does not travel alone and a "good Asian mother" does not leave her baby, although both are often required of INGO professionals. She argues this tension must arise because citizens of Asia are simply more family oriented than the individualistic peoples in the West. This tension is well known even at the top level of USFA, as the director, Ranny, cites not having kids as one of the reasons she was able to move into her position as director.

At USFA, no male worker expresses similar concerns about childcare or anxiety around travel, even though almost all male staff members have children. Male practitioners often describe traveling to the field as "inconvenient." They note "their families miss them," and sometimes they tell me they are concerned about their wife thinking they are cheating while traveling for work. Nevertheless, for male staff, it is assumed their female partner or parents will handle the childcare without difficulty in their absence. At lunch one day, Srey-na explains that although her husband is also a development worker, her in-laws do not shame him for traveling to the field or working at night like they do her. She sighs, "We are held to different standards . . . They tell me a good Cambodian mother should not be influenced by Western ideas about work."

Women all over the world frequently express difficulties combining work and family duties (Radhakrishnan and Solari 2023). In some ways, the problems Cambodian practitioners face are eerily similar to many American women's struggles to balance work and family in professional jobs, albeit in a very different cultural context. Nevertheless, despite similar difficulties with merging work and family in the U.S. context, female Khmer practitioners make sense of and resist their difficulties by juxtaposing their Asian experience with a Western one. This is particularly present in their descriptions of American female staff. USFA has two permanent American employees, the deputy director and a public health expert on the malaria team. Both are female. Often, Khmer workers point to these women, female visitors from headquarters, and even to me as examples of "Western" women who can travel easily to the field, "with no care for their families." The American USFA workers can also easily afford childcare in Phnom Penh on their expatriate salaries.

Srey-na reports that travel to the field can be fun, rewarding, and a chance to see how people really live in the countryside. However, travel is not easy for Cambodian women. "Asian women are expected to be with their families." In contrast, staff portray white women as unobligated by familial expectations and, by extension, lacking in family closeness or kinship networks. Khmer program manager Sovattha confronts Erin about this one day. Erin tells her she needs to go to the field to discuss their new project with the provincial health department staff. Sovattha directly challenges her, saying, "It is not as easy for me to go to the field, my parents will keep my children, but they will tell me the Western organization is making me a bad mother." Erin looks confused, explaining that both men and women go to the field at USFA and inquiring if her husband can keep her kids. Later, Sovattha complains to her coworker that this job is easy for Erin because she has a Cambodian nanny to take care of her two kids and she left her parents behind in the U.S.

When discussing such issues with me, Cambodian workers often inquire if I see these types of problems in Japanese INGOs. Dr. Belinda contends that if the women at USFA worked for a development organization with origins in Japan or South Korea they would not have issues combining work and family, as those organizations "understand Asian families." Nevertheless, when I ask them if they would prefer to work in a different sector, most women at USFA tell me development is a job where women have better opportunities to travel and move up to manager roles, particularly in the Western organizations. Sotheary explains that she came back to the capital to work at a USAID-funded organization because Western organizations are concerned about gender equality, and they want women to be strong.

Mother-workers at USFA struggle with the contradiction of having a workplace where gender equality rhetoric is highly valued and women can move up equally with men but, at the same time, of not having a workplace that addresses their unique needs due to caregiving expectations. Like Sotheary, female practitioners at USFA argue that their organization's leaders need to better understand the needs of Asian mothers, then find a middle ground between an Asian way and a Western one.

In the push for a hybrid middle ground, sometimes Cambodian worker-mothers do get managers to compromise. For instance, Chantrea makes a compelling case to Panh and Erin that the Western model of work must adapt to the Asian model of family. Panh helps her convince Erin to let Chantrea delay her field trips for two months until she has finished breast-feeding. Additionally, several USFA mothers proposed the idea of an onsite daycare or nursery to Ranny, who said she would consider it. Erin and Ranny were negotiating this request during my time at USFA, and a year later some stipends were provided for childcare for new moms. Chantrea and her coworkers celebrate these successes, telling me that eventually they believe managers will better understand the need to combine Western workplace equality with the demands of Asian motherhood. In this case, we see USFA staff use the notion of Asian families to address workplace inequalities faced by mother-workers. This creates a fairer work environment, solving some of the work-family conflicts that remain unsolved for many in the U.S. today.

However, not every attempt to resist gendered workplace inequalities was successful, and mothers cannot afford to opt out of the workforce and still maintain their urban, middle-class lifestyles. In these cases, they are pushed to leave their children with their grandparents, who frequently shame these mothers for doing so: hence the subtitle of this section, "The Grandparent Dilemma." In the U.S., it is assumed women will gain empowerment from entering the formal workforce, and the struggles of combining work and parenting are rarely addressed. At USFA, this problem unintentionally travels to the Cambodian context, where it is challenged by Khmer practitioners through the lens of Asian and Western imaginaries. Under USFA's model, Cambodian mothers interpret themselves as caught between being an ideal Western worker and an ideal Asian mother. However, not wanting to give up the opportunities afforded to them by USFA, they envision a future in which managers will increasingly hybridize Asian and Western ideas about gender and work.

Reinforcing and Resisting Work-Family Bargains

In this chapter we have seen that the donor gender regimes of Japan and the U.S. distinctly shape workplace inequalities at JSA and USFA. Yet these regimes are contested in organizational interactions. At JSA, we see Japanese practitioners resist their nation's gender regime while Khmer managers reinforce it. Khmer managers argue it is the "Asian way" to uphold "traditional" family norms and workplace gendered hierarchy. In contrast, at USFA, mother-workers try to resist workplace inequalities by contending that USFA's Western model needs to be combined with Asian motherhood. Cambodian worker-mothers envision a hybrid future where USFA will strike a compromise between Western workplace equality and Asian motherhood by providing benefits specifically geared towards new mothers. The distinctive meanings that "Asia" takes on in workplace interactions at JSA and USFA clearly illustrate the multivocality of the development imaginaries and the role they play in reworking beliefs about gender, work, and national advancement.

The findings here reveal that development takes place in deeply gendered workplaces. This impacts how development programming is implemented and practitioner experiences. As Cambodian practitioners employ schemas from the development imaginaries to make donor gender regimes meaningful in practice, practitioners sometimes produce outcomes that were not originally or explicitly intended by donors. Going further into workplace interactions, the next chapter documents how development imaginaries are used to make worker compensation meaningful in practice.

However, first it must be noted that the findings here can expand our understandings of gender in transnational workplaces more generally. Studies of transnational workplaces demonstrate that when organizations move their offices to a new country, they often reflect the institutional characteristics of their home countries in their operations abroad. Expatriate managers also bring their own gendered beliefs into management styles in transnational workplaces (Hart 2002; Helfen, Schüßler, and Stevis 2016; Wilks 2021; Lynch 2007). However, to be effective, transnational workplaces also need to adapt their operations to the new country's contexts. This process can result in "institutional dualism" or hybridization between home country and recipient country forces interacting to create new organizational strategies (Heidenreich 2012; Morgan and Kristensen 2006).

Additionally, "the vast feminist literature on globalization suggests that the material and ideological dimensions of motherhood are constructed, adopted, and contested in the context of the imperative for gendered subjects to work for wage" (Radhakrishnan 2022: 132). Consequently, meanings around motherhood and work are deeply intertwined as societies develop. Yet frequently gender regimes are studied only in the context of domestic state policies or institutions and compared cross-nationally (Giordano 2019). The cases of donor gender regimes and practitioners' modifications of them presented here illustrate the microlevel interactional processes through which gender regimes travel. Consequently, this chapter shows how transnational workplaces carry with them different solutions to the unequal burden of childcare, solutions which are hybridized in recipient nations. Examining how gender regimes travel and are adapted can provide new insights into the study, not just of foreign aid, but transnational workplaces more generally.

FIVE

Care Through Compensation
Patronage, Mistrust, and Transparency

At Japan Services Asia (JSA), Sovann tells me he has some frustrations with his Japanese bosses' compensation practices. Cambodian managers tell Japanese leadership about the importance of providing benefits like retreats, conference travel, or holiday gifts to Cambodian staff, but JSA does not provide them. He does not understand why Japanese managers provide extra benefits, like per diems, to state officials but will not do so for employees. Frustrated, Sovann asks if they know that "in Asia the boss must take care of the staff?"

In contrast, Srey-na works at U.S. Family Aid (USFA). She explains that to determine if you are working for a good employer, it is not just about what the job pays—most INGOs offer similar pay—it is really about the "extras" a job provides. If she was working for a bank, she would likely receive extra cash for her family on holidays, or if she had a government job, she could collect per diem payments. "NGOs can't do that, but they can *take care* of us in other ways." She reports that USFA provides benefits like meals, quality hotels during fieldwork, international travel opportunities, holiday gifts, parties, and staff retreats. "These types of benefits are how management shows workers that they truly value them [the workers] and their work. . . . For Cambodians . . . sometimes we want to see our employer almost like a patron."

As Sovann and Srey-na's comments illustrate, in Cambodia, patronage is not just a political system, it is also a cultural schema workers utilize to understand their relationship to their employers. This chapter examines JSA and USFA's budgeting and compensation practices along with the benefits each INGO provides. As we know from previous chapters, Japan's gender regime prioritizes upgrading the capacity of public health officials to improve women's health services. Consequently, JSA has a budget for paying per diem to state officials but does not have a budget for extra staff benefits. In contrast, USFA's donors emphasize the need to support civil society and the private sector. To do so, USAID maintains funds for building the capacity of Cambodian employees as members of civil society.

Next, the chapter investigates workplace interactions in which Cambodian staff use the development imaginaries to make JSA and USFA's financial practices meaningful within patronage expectations. Encountering these two distinctive gender regimes and budget practices, INGO managers engage in "relational work" or "the creative effort people make establishing, maintaining, negotiating, transforming, and terminating interpersonal relations around money" (Zelizer 2012: 149). Relational work draws attention to how interpersonal interactions shape the accomplishment of economic exchanges.

Relational work is often necessary to frame compensation in a way that is meaningful to those receiving it. For instance, Almeling (2007) finds workers at egg and sperm banks carefully frame financial exchange differently based on a client's gender. Egg donors were told they were providing a gift to expectant parents, but sperm donors were said to be engaging in paid labor. Relational work can be done to make economic exchange meaningful, determine the level of trust around the exchange, and generate satisfaction or dissatisfaction with compensation and exchange partners.

When compensation does not take the right form, relationships are strained, and when employees and employers disagree on financial meanings, workers may see employers as unworthy exchange partners. This can lead workers to resist employers, disengage, or try to find new employment (Mears 2015). As we will see below, relational work in each INGO is done by foreign and Cambodian managers, often utilizing the development imaginaries to make financial practices meaningful. Relational work plays a key role in whether the staff of each INGO see their organization's leadership as worthy exchange partners or "good patrons." However, before evaluating compensation and relational work in each INGO, I briefly examine the history of patronage in Cambodia, alongside its ties to masculinity.

Patronage and Masculinity in Cambodia

As we saw in Sovann and Srey-na's stories, Cambodians make sense of compensation through the lens of "patronage." In Cambodia, "patronage, alliances and networks remain an integral part of everyday life" (Jacobsen 2008: 138). The term "patronage" is used by participants to describe political networks, such as government officials practicing vote buying, as well as power networks not directly linked to political parties (although most are), like influential community members providing money to those with fewer resources (Hutchcroft 2014). The latter practice is sometimes referred to as "clientelism," where "persons of higher social status (patrons) are linked to those of lower social status (clients) in face-to-face ties of reciprocity that can vary in content and purpose across time" (Hutchcroft 2014: 54).

Cambodians have organized social relations via patronage practices and kinship networks for over a thousand years (Jacobsen and Stuart-Fox 2013). Before the founding of the Angkor Empire (800–1300 AD) in rural Cambodia, it is believed that power relations in farming villages were organized around families and kinship groups, with important community leaders establishing themselves as patrons (Chandler 2007). Once the Angkor Empire was established, central government figures constructed extensive patronage networks. Acting as patrons to local administrators in rural communities throughout the empire, patronage was a crucial element of Angkorian politics (Mabbett 1977). Patron-client power relations lasted through both French colonization and the brutal Khmer Rouge regime, although not without adaptation. Currently, despite the efforts of international organizations to impart the importance of democracy and transparent governance to Cambodians, the dominant political party, the Cambodian People's Party (CPP), continues to maintain power largely through patronage networks (Jacobsen and Stuart-Fox 2013).

Strong cultural beliefs around social hierarchy in Cambodia legitimize patronage, enabling it to endure throughout regime changes. Within minutes of meeting each other, Cambodians can establish where they fit in the social hierarchy in relation to the others present on the basis of "age, sex, familial background, birth order, occupation, political position, influence, education, personal character, and financial benevolence" (Jacobsen and Stuart-Fox 2013: 9). In Cambodia, social hierarchy is justified through the Buddhist belief that people who are born in high positions acquired *bunn*, or merit, in a past life, giving them a moral right to their high social standing. Moreover, the population's memory of the Khmer Rouge and political turmoil in the recent past, puts a high value on maintaining a stable social order. These cultural and political forces make it difficult to challenge those who hold wealth and power or change the patronage system more generally (Jacobsen and Stuart-Fox 2013).

Additionally, success in the patronage system is frequently associated with masculinity (Jacobsen 2011). Throughout modern history, it has largely been men who have enacted the role of patrons and powerful leaders in Cambodia (Frieson 2001; Jacobsen 2008). Successful masculinity is associated with wealth, modern dress, caring for your family and kinship networks, and powerful positions (Jacobsen 2011). Becoming a successful man nearly always requires participating in patronage networks and reliance on a more powerful patron for opportunities. In contrast, cultural norms that push women into the private sphere often make it more difficult for them to participate in patronage systems. The few women who have achieved political power are often those who were born into politically powerful families with preexisting patronage networks (Jacobsen and Stuart-Fox 2013).

In Cambodia, foreign aid donors and INGOs have been integrated into existing patronage systems (Ear 2013). For instance, politicians frequently portray themselves as the patrons who have attracted foreign aid projects. Due to this legacy, it is not unexpected that the Cambodian development sector faces strong donor demands for financial transparency in an attempt to counter what donors assume are the "corrupt financial practices" embedded in a patronage system. However, Cambodians themselves use the term "patronage" in complex, and sometimes conflicting, ways. Frequently patronage is used to describe corrupt financial practices or dishonesty in the political system. Yet it is also a dominant cultural schema through which Cambodians interpret economic exchange and employer-employee relationships.

Like Srey-na and Sovann, many Khmer workers assume a good employer is one that can "give generous gifts" and "take care of them." Many Cambodians maintain the assumption that financial caretaking is the Asian way of doing business. In doing so, they draw on a larger association with gift-giving, opacity, and patronage in Asian financial practices (Hoang 2018; Kim 2017). Consequently, employers in Cambodia are expected to provide not just basic monetary compensation for the job but also nonmonetary benefits or gifts to be seen as worthy exchange partners or good patrons. Below, I investigate first how each INGO's donor gender regime and financial practices impact its compensation practices. Then I analyze how patronage expectations are interpreted through relational work at Japanese Services Asia and U.S. Family Aid.

Japan Services Asia's Financial Practices

Budgeting and compensation practices at Japan Services Asia (JSA) are impacted by two key aspects of Japan's gender regime and JICA's financial management policies. The first aspect is Japan's focus on the state's capacity to provide women's health services. The emphasis on state capacity means that the portion of JICA's budget that goes to building the managerial and technical skills of Cambodians—its "capacity-building budget"—goes to paying state officials per diems or providing officials with extra trainings and benefits. As we saw in chapter 2, these practices mean JSA is seen as a worthy exchange partner or "good patron" by state officials. Yet this practice left limited funds to compensate workers with extra benefits.

Second, JSA's gendered work context modified the meaning of compensation for the organization. As detailed in chapter 4, JSA's hiring practices are a result of both Japan's labor market legacy and the Cambodian context. JSA hires only male program managers to facilitate interactions with male state officials. Managers are expected to focus their energy on implementing project activities in cooperation with state officials. At the same time, Japanese managers are largely women. As we will see below, these hiring practices shape the way that JSA's compensation is interpreted by Japanese and Cambodian staff.

Finally, JSA's financial policies are further impacted by JICA's budgeting and financial management practices. JICA places less emphasis on budget transparency than USAID, which may, in part, be due to lower levels of professionalization in Japan's nonprofit and NGO sector. Due to its emphasis on the developmental state, Japan's nonprofit and NGO sector developed much later than the U.S.'s and is strictly separated from the private sector. The limited number of nonprofits and NGOs in Japan prior to the 1980s is attributed to Japan's strong "developmental state" characterized by the "Iron Triangle," a tight collaboration of ruling party, corporations, and powerful bureaucracy. This collaboration, with the capacity for long-term economic planning, dedicated itself to Japan's rapid industrialization. It left little space for interest groups to be heard by the government or participate in the market (Hirata 2002; Reimann 2010). It was not until the late 1980s

that economic downturn, rising fiscal deficit, and several political corruption scandals sowed seeds of doubt in the developmental state (Hirata
2002). Additionally, until 1998, Japanese regulatory structures made it very
difficult to register as a "public interest" organization in Japan. In consequence, Japan has a limited nonprofit sector compared to other industrialized democracies (Pekkanen 2006; Reimann 2010).

In the 1980s, alongside the domestic economic downturn that lessened
faith in Japan's development state, several factors pressured Japan to rethink its nonprofit and NGO sector. First, "the Indochina refugee crisis"
was highly publicized in Japan. Japanese citizens were deeply concerned
by the humanitarian crisis taking place in Southeast Asia and the growing
number of Cambodian refugees in camps on the Thai-Cambodia border.
Numerous voluntary groups emerged in Japan to care for refugees in Thailand and Cambodia (Hirata 2002). Japanese foreign aid also faced criticism from the international community for its strong emphasis on loans,
infrastructure, and technical assistance and limited support for "soft" aid
(Reimann 2010). While Japan has long been a generous development donor,
Japanese development assistance traditionally focused on government-to-
government grants and loans. Finally, in 1995, Japan confronted the Great
Hanshin-Awaji Earthquake, which acted as a catalyst for increasing public
approval of the nonprofit sector (Osborne 2003). The government was slow
to act in response to this crisis, but volunteer groups rushed to help. The
work of relief organizations in response to the earthquake was highly publicized (Pekkanen 2000; Yamashita 2012).

In response to these international and domestic factors, Japan's Ministry of Foreign Affairs set up its first grant program for INGOs in 1989.
By 1999, Japan had liberalized its nonprofit and NGO laws. After this, the
number of nonprofits and NGOs in the country increased rapidly. Nevertheless, due to this late development, Japan's INGO sector is smaller and
less professionalized in comparison to many of its counterparts in the West.
JICA has continued to develop its budgeting and monitoring regulations
for INGOs over the years, yet its regulations are not nearly as arduous as
USAID's. Consequently, there is not the same level of pressure for financial
transparency for JICA projects.

As a result, at JSA, the JICA budget is private and all Khmer staff members, except one, are unaware of how much the budget is in total or how it is
allocated. As we will see, this is in stark contrast to U.S. Family Aid, where
transparency around the budget for all staff members is mandated. This

reliance on personal relations in project design and organizational finances may stem from Japan's business culture, in which personal relationships were traditionally a key part of successful economic interactions (Hutchcroft 2014; Whitley 1991).

During her visit to the Cambodia office from Tokyo, I had the opportunity to speak with a JSA headquarters staff member, Emiko. Before taking the position at headquarters, Emiko worked at JICA. I ask her why JSA does not tell any staff members how much money is in the JICA grant. She explains frankly that she thinks it is very unfortunate, but "JICA does not trust the local people to implement or with money." She believes they should spend more on local workers than they do, since JSA is making a big difference by building the skills of local workers. "But, for JICA, they don't know them, and they don't trust them."

With a more limited demand for financial transparency, reduced trust for local workers, and an emphasis on social ties, JSA practiced private budgeting. The only employees at JSA who ever saw the full project budget were Japanese staff members and one Khmer accountant who had worked for the organization for over fifteen years. Financial decisions were often made in conversations between JICA representatives, JSA headquarters staff, and Japanese managers from the Cambodia office. Other than the accountant, all Khmer staff members at JSA were charged with project implementation duties. JSA's emphasis on state capacity, gendered hiring practices, and private budgeting practices all shape relational work at JSA.

Relational Work at Japan Services Asia

While at first glance, one might assume these personalistic relations around money would be a better fit with Cambodia's patronage system, private budgeting at Japan Services Asia (JSA) breeds a culture of mistrust around finances between Cambodian and Japanese staff. At the JSA office in Steung Treng, I am assisting a program assistant, Chea, with her English vocabulary. She tells me she asked her manager, Sovann, why JSA staff do not have a holiday party. He said that the Japanese bosses do not care about the workers at JSA. She looks worried and says she wants to improve her skills in English in case she needs to get a different job.

At JSA, Japanese and Cambodian managers engage in relational work to define the meaning of employee-employer economic exchange. The concept of relational work is not solely about the concrete resources provided through economic exchange, but it also draws attention to the negotiated meanings or framings around economic exchange (Bandelj 2020; Zelizer 2012). As we will see below, Japanese and Cambodian managers at JSA engage in divergent framings of compensation. Japanese managers try to generate employee satisfaction with compensation. Yet Cambodian managers work against Japanese staff to frame JSA's compensation practices as limited. Workplace interactions around finances typically revolve around three aspects: budgeting, reporting, and compensation.

PRIVATE BUDGETING

At JSA, all Cambodian staff members except one are unaware of how much the budget is in total or how it is allocated. Budget documents are also written in Japanese. This means Cambodian managers focus solely on project activities and state relationships in their jobs. In consequence, Cambodian managers did not have an opportunity to weigh in on staff benefits at JSA. Moreover, Cambodian staff are often mistrusted when it comes to money. Samnang's story below introduces the tensions that arise from privacy around budgeting at JSA.

After a tense staff meeting about employee benefits, I'm riding back to Phnom Penh with JSA's program manager, Samnang. We drive down dirt roads, passing rural villages and rice farms. He is telling me about the tarps filled with rice laid out on the ground in front of many of the farms we are driving by. Rice farmers lay the rice out to dry after it has been harvested. In this process, farmers often enlist the help of chickens to walk on the rice and separate it so it will dry more quickly, preventing mildew. Samnang points out the numerous chickens walking on the rice-covered tarps, pecking at the ground.

He goes on to say, as the chicken is walking it sneaks a few bites of rice here and there because the rice is also the chicken's food. He then exclaims that the story is a metaphor. "This is like corruption, you see . . . when people have to deal with money, they cannot help but *see* a little bit too." (See is the Khmer word for "eat" that is used to describe animals, but not humans, eating. However, *see loi*, or "eat money," is also a slang way of talking about corruption in Cambodia). Samnang goes on, saying that he knows Cambodians can be like this, but people from other countries can be too.

He says that he believes there is some "small corruption" at JSA among Cambodian staff. Often, when staff buy workshop materials or snacks at the market, they might pocket a few extra dollars. Other coworkers might ask the gas station attendant to change the receipt so they can keep a few dollars to themselves. He wishes he did not have to deal with money at all at JSA due to these issues. However, he starts to get more heated talking about the Japanese staff, stating that "they make these problems much worse." Samnang is angry his Japanese managers treat expatriates, even me, as immediately trustworthy with money while mistrusting Cambodians. In a heated voice, he asks, "What is a few dollars here and there?"

Instead, what he tells me is that what he is really mistrustful of—is the Japanese staff's privacy about money. Samnang explicates, "sometimes people come to change Cambodia but then Cambodia changes you." His father's friend from JICA told him about a Japanese woman who came to Cambodia as an NGO director and then ran off to another country with her organization's money. In a suspicious tone, he reports he does not know what Junko and Hanako are doing because they are so private about money. "It could happen here." I saw absolutely no evidence that any of the Japanese staff at JSA are corrupt. Nevertheless, to Samnang, since they are mistrustful about financial reporting and not providing extra benefits to the staff, he presumes Japanese managers must be keeping those benefits for themselves.

Samnang interprets JSA's privacy around budgeting through the lens of patronage, generating mistrust around economic exchange at JSA. As a result, Cambodian managers often framed JSA's Japanese managers as "suspicious" or unworthy exchange partners. This suspicion that arose from private budgeting made it difficult for Japanese managers to recruit local managers to undertake cooperative relational work, helping Japanese staff make compensation and reporting practices palatable to staff. Private budgeting sets the stage for tension around reporting and compensation at JSA.

REPORTING

Private budgeting creates an environment for mistrustful reporting and receipt-writing interactions at JSA. Like most NGO practitioners, JSA's staff face obligations to carefully report how much money their organization spent and how they spent it. JSA hosts workshops for public health officials and villagers, all of which require Cambodian staff to fill out financial reports. Additionally, JSA staff write receipts for per diems provided to public health workers. JSA managers who live in Phnom Penh on weekends also need to write receipts more frequently than USFA staff to be reimbursed for weekly travel. Yet, unlike at USFA, where, as we will see below, receipts and reporting are understood to be part of the job, JSA staff do not have a work background in other international development organizations and thus a culture of seemingly endless receipts and financial reporting is new for them.

In addition, receipts are strictly checked by the director and accountant. JSA's director, Junko, believes that staff are always trying to "sneak away with a few dollars." Junko is suspicious about staff receipts. She often cross-checks the costs of items by going back to the market to inquire with sellers how much workers paid for workshop materials or food items. In the process of receipt checking, JSA's Khmer accountant, Atith, is often put in the middle. Junko urges him to check every dollar spent. In Junko's absence, program managers tell Atith that the Cambodian staff should all be on the same side. The managers question if he believes workers deserve more benefits and tell him to make that case with Junko. Atith plays both sides. He follows up on receipts as Junko requests, telling managers it is not his fault, he is just doing what Junko says. Yet at staff meetings, he sides with managers, advocating for better staff benefits.

Trust in local staff is limited to such a degree that when JSA's accountant, Atith, takes a leave of absence, Junko and her Japanese intern, Hanako, request that I be the one to fill in for him and help with basic accounting. They taught me to add the daily expenditures to the budget, check receipts, and dole out needed cash to employees. They translate budgeting lines from Japanese to English for me. When I inquire why another staff member does not fill in, Junko explains it is not ideal that I am doing the accounting since I am just a volunteer, but it is better that a foreigner does it than local staff. To everyone's relief, the accountant returned just a couple weeks later, as my skills in accounting turn out to be quite limited.

Receipts and financial reporting are a source of frequent frustration at JSA. This frustration is directly framed as the fault of Japanese managers by Cambodian staff. Program manager Boran complains that Japanese managers count every dollar Cambodian staff spend, but they do not tell us where the rest of the money is going. On a rare day, Junko and Hanako are at a JICA meeting in Phnom Penh and staff are left alone at the office. Boran shows staff a video about USAID accounting practices and transparency. In uncommon praise for the West, after watching the video, JSA's Khmer staff discuss the fact that NGO workers at organizations funded by the U.S. must know more about the budget than they do. Several staff members ask me if I think this is true. Boran stokes staff suspicion by asking them to consider the question—Why are other NGOs transparent about their budgets, but not JSA? Private budgeting practices and mistrust surrounding receipt-writing feed Khmer workers' assumptions that Japanese managers—and therefore JSA—is a suspicious patron. Contributing to this tension is disagreement over how workers should be compensated.

RESISTING COMPENSATION

Following JICA's logic in prioritizing state officials' capacity, limited attention is given to upgrading the skills of staff members at JSA. This means the JICA budget provides salaries for staff but limited extra benefits, since there is not a capacity-building budget for INGO staff. In terms of compensation, JSA and USFA employees make relatively similar salaries. JSA does provide staff with compensated meals, fieldwork, and holiday parties, although on a smaller scale than USFA. Additionally, it provides one opportunity for international travel to Japan for staff who have worked for JSA for more than five years. However, it does not provide perks like holiday giveaways, frequent international travel for workshops, fancy hotels for fieldwork, or cash extras for staff, which USFA and many other INGOs do.

But JSA did provide rather expansive medical and education benefits for workers and their children that USFA did not. These funds support up to 200 US dollars per year in medical spending and financed after-school education programs for employees' children. One visitor from headquarters presented these benefits as gifts, telling staff that education and health benefits are essential for "citizens of Asia." She draws on the idea that, across Asia, children are sent to after-school programs to upgrade their education, a practice common in China, Japan, Singapore, and South Korea. This relational work on the part of Japanese staff uses regional rhetoric in a clear effort to frame compensation practices as appealing.

This framing of JSA's compensation practices is largely ignored. Embedded in a culture of organizational distrust, Japanese managers are not successful in enlisting the cooperation of Khmer managers in framing staff compensation as acceptable. As we will see below, in USFA's case, Cambodian managers help foreign managers frame activities like travel and meal per diems as gifts from USFA. Collaboration between Cambodian and foreign managers in relational work enables local managers to explain the cultural meanings of money in Cambodia to foreign managers. However, without the assistance of Cambodian managers in framing compensation,

Japanese managers struggle to articulate to Cambodian workers that their health and education benefits are gifts from their employer.

Cambodian managers also directly work against Japanese managers by engaging in relational work that frames JSA's worker compensation as limited. Sovann rejects the regional rhetoric of Japanese managers through inter-Asian comparisons. Sovann tells two program assistants that Japanese managers lived in "rich Japan" too long, so they do not know how to provide holiday parties or giveaways. Sovann says his cousin told him that Chinese and Singaporean businessmen always do these types of things for their employees. Khmer managers also tell staff that medical and education resources are just basic benefits in a professional job. Additionally, after-school programs are largely held in Phnom Penh and often unavailable to the children of many rural staff members. Thus, Japanese managers are largely unsuccessful in their attempts to frame the medical and educational benefits JSA provides to fit the logic of patronage.

The failure of Japanese managers to frame compensation appropriately is surprising given the fact that regional rhetoric about Asian cultural similarity is often an incredibly effective tool for legitimizing the work of JSA. We have seen regional similarity used successfully in numerous other cases presented in this book's chapters. Additionally, Japan itself has a legacy of patronage politics, which one might have thought would enable them to better understand Cambodians' cultural meanings around money (Reed 2021). Yet studies have also illustrated that Japan's legacy of a high-stress work ethic does not always transfer well to other Southeast Asian nations (Kamal et al. 2020). In JSA's case, we see Cambodian managers working against Japanese managers in framing employee compensation, validating the financial practices of both the West and other East Asian nations to do so. This makes it very difficult for Japanese managers to be understood as worthy exchange partners by their Cambodian employees.

At JSA, compensation framing tensions are also impacted by the organization's gendered hiring practices, creating a situation in which beliefs about gender difference trump Asian similarity rhetoric. One day, two female headquarters staff members are visiting, and a staff meeting about employee benefits takes place. There, Samnang demands to know why JSA supports per diems and travel benefits for government officials but will not have a retreat for staff. The headquarters staff members look at one another confused, as this proposal is clearly foreign to them; one inquires, "Where would the budget for that come from?" Yet male Cambodian managers draw on gendered norms that link masculinity to patronage politics, interpreting Japanese managers' resistance to doing things like providing staff retreats or gifts as evidence of the fact that "women are bad patrons."

As discussed in chapter 2, on several occasions, Junko tries to say officials should not need per diem to do their jobs. Managers argue with her, explaining that per diem is the way things are done in Cambodia. Samnang brings up the fact that managers have had to remind Junko to continue to pay per diem to state officials as further evidence for the idea that Japanese women are bad patrons. He argues that Japanese women just do not understand the way things are done. Japan is too rich now. In this case, the fact that Japan was the first East Asian nation to industrialize is used to argue that Japanese managers are out of touch with the rest of Asia. Sovann also contends women are bad patrons because they rarely work in the private sector. He explains there are not many female businesswomen in Japan or in Phnom Penh. This lack of experience in the private sector means women do not know that Asian employers must show their workers appreciation through gifts and parties.

Program managers frequently complain to other staff about limited compensation at JSA. On the same day staff watch the USAID budgeting video discussed above, Cambodian managers have all staff watch a video about a well-known Western INGO and its worker benefits. They argue that Western organizations know better how to appreciate their workers, suddenly praising the practices of INGOs from Europe, the U.S., and Australia, which they frequently disparage. Financial practices are the only aspect in which I see Khmer managers at JSA use the development imaginary of the West to resist at JSA.

As we saw in Samnang's metaphor about chickens and rice farming, JSA's private budgeting style, mistrustful relationships around reporting, and the lack of culturally expected benefits cause workers to be suspicious of (particularly female) Japanese managers. This constrains Japanese managers from enlisting Cambodian managers to collaborate in the relational work needed to frame compensation practices to fit employees' patronage expectations. Japanese managers are left to make JSA seem like a worthy exchange partner alone, attempting to appease Cambodian managers and employees. Without the necessary cultural knowledge, Japanese managers are unsuccessful in adapting their financial practices to the Cambodian context. This lack of success is also due, in large part, to the fact that Cambodian managers often engage in relational work that actively frames the benefits Japanese managers provide as lacking. In consequence, JSA is interpreted by Cambodian workers as an unworthy exchange partner or "bad patron."

U.S. Family Aid's Financial Practices

The U.S. gender regime and its financial practices also modify the way relational work takes place at U.S. Family Aid (USFA). First, the U.S. gender regime prioritizes building the capacity of the private sector and nongovernmental organizations to upgrade women's health, as discussed earlier. The U.S.'s long history of nonprofit organizing leads it to have large and highly professionalized nonprofit and NGO sectors (Skocpol, Ganz, and Munson 2000). After the American Revolution, the early American state found taxation and service provision difficult to implement, leading to a rise in nonprofit service provision. Throughout the 1800s, Christian charities and religious organizations provided nonprofit services such as education, healthcare, orphanages, and eldercare (Hammack 2002).

After 1960, another wave of nonprofit expansion occurred for several reasons. First, American affluence continued to grow. Americans could increasingly afford to purchase services from and provide support to nonprofit organizations, such as private education or patronage of the arts. Second, the Great Society programs enacted by President Lyndon Johnson increased subsidies to nonprofits. Third, nonprofits were involved in the wave of mobilization in this era, including the Civil Rights Movement and the anti–Vietnam War movement (Hammack 2002). Finally, in 1969, the Tax Reform Act further liberalized charitable organization status and tax exemptions for donors. With these changes, nonprofits were provided with the opportunity to act as influential interest groups and partners to the American state.

Additionally, when USAID was established in the 1960s, there was a movement against big government and bureaucracy. This pushed USAID to subgrant to INGOs as nonprofit actors to provide services abroad early on in its aid programming (Krause 2014). By the 1980s, nonprofits and NGOs were referred to as the "third sector" in the U.S., providing ample employment opportunities. Currently, the nonprofit sector comprises an estimated 5 percent of the GDP in the U.S. (Indiana Nonprofits Project 2017). Historically, the U.S. government itself has been a generous donor to the sector.

Although USAID does not publish the exact number, scholars estimate that before its closing approximately 28 percent of USAID's aid budget (which was nearly 43 billion in 2024) was funneled through INGOs (Tarnoff and Lawson 2016). For comparison, this is much more than most developed nations, such as Britain, where about 5 percent of bilateral funding goes to INGOs (Stroup 2012). INGO practitioners in the U.S. are deemed legitimate development experts and provided with numerous opportunities to cooperate with government agencies.

Given the well-funded, professionalized nonprofit sector in its own country, USAID exports this model by focusing on upgrading the skills of INGO workers. For this reason, it provides a capacity-building budget for NGO staff. At USFA, community members in need of health services are consider the "primary" beneficiaries of the USAID project. Then, INGO workers are considered the "secondary" beneficiaries of the project. USAID considers upgrading the skills of NGO workers as an essential part of promoting civil society in Cambodia. This means USAID supplies a budget for staff development while, as we saw in chapter 2, providing government official per diems is strictly forbidden.[1] Cambodian managers also have partial say in how the staff capacity-building budget is spent.

Second, as we have seen, the U.S. gender regime fosters very different hiring practices than those of JSA. USAID demands USFA promote gender equality through multiple methods, including NGO hiring practices. USAID promotes the hiring of male and female employees at nearly equal rates when possible. USFA is also pushed to hire female managers when it can. USFA's director is a well-respected Khmer woman, Ranny. While the deputy director, a program manager, and the chief of party are all foreignborn, the rest of the managers at USFA are Cambodian and all but one are women.

With its Cambodian director and managers, USFA empowers Cambodians, particularly its director, Ranny, to have influence over foreign-born managers. For instance, Erin looks to Ranny and other Khmer managers to explain to her how best to reward staff, particularly when it comes to using the capacity-building budget. This empowers Cambodian staff to assist foreign-born managers in framing USFA's financial practices to fit the patronage expectations of Cambodian staff.

Finally, in terms of donor financial practices, transparent budgeting is a high priority for USAID (or was until recently). In the U.S., the nonprofit and private sectors are not strongly distinguished, meaning management and budgeting techniques from the private sector are often used in INGOs. U.S.-based INGOs are expected to demonstrate financial transparency and efficacy in the use of funding (Stroup 2012). For instance, the following statement is presented by FHI360, a large USAID-funded health INGO headquartered in Washington, D.C., in its guidebook for acquiring funding from USAID:

> As a steward of USAID funds, one of your goals is to make sure your organization uses this money appropriately and effectively to deliver needed services to beneficiaries. The procurement regulations are meant to ensure that funds are not mismanaged or used to purchase dangerous or low-quality goods that could cause more harm than good. Establishing an appropriate procurement process helps protect your organization and beneficiaries, promotes transparency and accountability, and helps ensure that funds are used efficiently to deliver needed services (FHI360 2010: 34).

As FHI360's example shows, there was a strong demand for transparency and high reliance on metrics for any INGO that worked with USAID. These financial practices have important consequences on relational work around budgeting and reporting at USFA.

Relational Work at U.S. Family Aid

One day, monitoring and evaluation specialist Chantrea and I sit chatting in our cubicle in USFA's Phnom Penh office. She tells me she thinks Director Ranny—or, as many staff members call her, "Madam" Ranny—is really smart. Chantrea explains that Ranny knows how to get the Western donors and foreigners to compensate Cambodian workers in a way that make sense in Asia. When I inquire further, Chantrea tells me Ranny knows how to follow the rules of the West, but she also can help foreign managers "take care" of USFA staff.

Although USFA and Japan Services Asia staff do not make drastically different salaries, they do receive different types of benefits. Additionally, budgeting and compensation are framed differently by managers at each organization. As we start to see in Chantrea's description, at USFA, Director Ranny and other Cambodian managers hybridize Western and Asian imaginaries to "take care" of Cambodian staff. They do so through workplace interactions around the same three aspects: budgeting, reporting, and compensation.

TRANSPARENT BUDGETING

In a large conference room, USFA staff meet with their private sector partner, DataFirst, the organization helping them conduct research and branding workshops on health behavior change for their USAID project. The staff of both organizations are going over a presentation they will be giving at an upcoming conference. Things start to get tense as DataFirst's expatriate staff member, Brigette, disapproves of the fact that her Khmer DataFirst colleague and a USFA practitioner are presenting the data together. She says DataFirst was hired to collect this data, and they must be the one to present that work product. They also must brand it with the DataFirst logo. USFA staff members contend this is a shared project that they also worked hard on. In response, Brigette raises her voice, "You know how important transparency is for USAID. We were budgeted to do this work product, my staff worked hard on it, and we need to be the ones to present it."

Illustrating the blurry line between the private and nonprofit sector, USFA staff and their organizational partners are careful about budget transparency and intellectual property rights. American managers at USFA contend that, when it comes to how their USAID money is used, there can be "no secrets" and "everyone knows where it goes." USFA's American deputy director, Erin, often reminds workers of the need for complete budget transparency and "no funny business" to remain competitive for USAID grants. Erin clearly interprets economic exchange to be impersonal, making statements like "money isn't personal" and that it is her job to ensure budget transparency because that is "how good business is done."

Following this insistence on transparency, all staff members at USFA are aware of how much money USAID provided for this project. Staff often examine the predetermined budget on a large screen in full staff meetings, and workers are aware of how much money is available for each activity. This enables Ranny, Erin, and other USFA managers to be clear with all staff members about how much money is in the budget and where it goes. This practice enables trust as there is no part of the budget staff are not privy to and everyone knows how each budget line will be used.

Furthermore, when it is time to disperse the staff capacity-building budget and design staff activities, American managers, like Deputy Director Erin, look to Director Ranny and other Cambodian managers to explain to her how best to reward Cambodian staff for working hard. Cambodian managers convince American ones to strategically use a portion of the staff capacity budget to provide what Cambodian workers would see as "patronage" benefits, such as dinners out, extra cash when traveling for fieldwork, and free giveaways during holidays.

This meant that the capacity-building budget enabled USFA managers to actually provide a few extra benefits of a nature that would be considered appropriate compensation for Cambodian employees under the cultural expectations of patronage. As American managers are able to enlist the assistance of Cambodian managers in the distribution of the staff capacity resources, they are better able to fit workers' patronage expectations when it comes to reporting and compensation.

REPORTING

After reviewing poorly written travel expenditure reports one too many times, a headquarters employee from Washington, D.C., Britney, gives USFA's staff an expenditure reporting training. She carefully reviews the well-documented protocols for submitting reports and tells staff that she knows this is annoying, but we must follow USAID's exact requirements to keep our funding going. This is how USAID confirms that no funds are being mismanaged.

Like JSA staff, USFA employees are required to engage in ample financial reporting. USFA workers often lament the mandate of "never-ending paperwork" to keep their USAID grant. All workers fill out receipts for travel to the field, workshop purchases, consultant contracts, and so on. Staff know that everything must be carefully accounted for when it comes to the USAID budget. Nevertheless, since they did not travel to and from Phnom Penh every week, like JSA staff did, receipt writing is a slightly smaller portion of the everyday labor of most USFA staff. Most of the budgeting and accounting work is done by a single Khmer accountant who is in charge of budget reporting. He made short budget reports at monthly staff meetings about how USFA is doing on spending the USAID grant.

However, for the financial reporting that staff are required to do at USFA, Cambodian and American managers cooperate to frame annoying financial reporting requirements, not as mandated by on-site managers, but as the fault of distant bureaucrats in Washington, D.C. A Cambodian manager, Panh, explains to Erin it is important to make sure staff know these budgeting practices are coming from the higher-ups and "people in your country, not us." Then they can see that here, in Cambodia, managers trust staff. Erin agrees to engage in the rhetoric that blames budgeting practices as incoming from far-away bureaucrats in the West. Consequently, managers work together to push blame for the annoying number of reporting requirements entailed in transparency budgeting onto USAID and the development imaginary of the West more generally. Such collaboration is enabled by U.S.-mandated transparency budgeting, as Cambodian managers did know exactly how the budget would be used and could explain to staff why financial reporting is necessary to make sure the budget is spent correctly.

During my observation at USFA, I overhear Chantrea's manager come to tell her she submitted the wrong receipt paperwork from a recent trip to the field. He tells her she will have to do it again because "you know how the donors are." She rolls her eyes and sighs as he walks away. She turns to commiserate with her coworker, Sokmy, about the annoyance of this requirement, saying "USAID and the other donors from Europe and Australia always ask too much, why is the system like this?" Yet, when staff are annoyed by reporting requirements, they do not blame USFA's managers. Instead, they blame distant others in Washington D.C. Essentially, at USFA, the cultural difference of distant bosses in the West and Cambodian practitioners is used to justify financial practices that would not have been acceptable under patronage. In consequence, unlike what we saw at JSA, staff do not perceive reporting requirements to be the personal fault of USFA's managers.

HYBRIDIZING COMPENSATION

While workers bristle against Western donor financial reporting requirements, Ranny and other Cambodian managers are careful to frame USFA's compensation practices and benefits in a way that fits staff patronage expectations. On the final workday before the Khmer New Year holiday, USFA staff members work a half-day. After lunch, workers excitedly change into traditional clothing for USFA's annual Khmer New Year party. USFA's outdoor area is elaborately decorated, traditional dancers are hired, the event is catered, alcohol is provided, and a stage is set up. There are talent contests and a raffle for employees to win home appliances, USFA-branded shirts, and cash prizes. After the contests, we eat, drink, and chat at large tables set up outside. Finally, we dance and sing as a DJ's music plays over the sound system. On the dance floor, USFA worker Sokmy yells to me over the music "these are the perks of working here" and then raises his beer as if to say "Cheers!"

Using the capacity-building budget allowance, Cambodian managers do carefully plan elaborate team-building retreats and holiday gatherings. However, Cambodian managers can only provide some extra benefits through this budget. Largely, relational work is done to strategically shape staff perceptions of the benefits that USFA can provide. Cambodian managers at USFA portray meals, conferences, and fieldwork travel opportunities as benefits to staff from their patron, USFA. When one program coordinator is annoyed about a deadline, Ranny reminds her she went to Washington, D.C., last year because USFA "is good to her."

In another example, at a meeting, staff member Kunthea is rewarded for her excellent reporting practices with a trip to Bangkok for a workshop. Ranny tells the staff that USFA is "good to those who work hard" as a few other staff members ask Kunthea to bring them back items from Bangkok. This is bolstered by the familiar and friendly environment in which staff work, often calling each other bong, or sibling, instead of by formal titles. By carefully creating a familial environment and framing INGO activities like conference meals and fieldwork hotels as extra perks, Ranny succeeds in setting up USFA, and herself, in a patron role. This role is what is expected by Cambodian staff to perceive their employer as a worthy exchange partner. Staff frequently discuss this through the Asian development imaginary, arguing that, even though they work for Western donors, Ranny and other Cambodian managers know that in Asia employers take good care of employees.

American managers lean on US market logic to explain why they give Cambodian managers leeway in how staff capacity funds should be spent and framed. They believe Cambodian managers better understand what Cambodian workers expect and that providing the appropriate benefits is good for business by helping USFA stay competitive. At the Khmer New Year party, Erin explains that the party might seem over the top, but this is just what companies do for workers in Cambodia. She tells me USFA must be able to compete with other places where Cambodian staff could work. Here we see competitive hiring used as the rationale for engaging with patronage compensation practices for employees.

Still, this American and Cambodian manager alliance sometimes requires Cambodian managers to override American ones. Sitting just outside the USFA director's office, I overhear Erin ask Ranny why she is letting so many staff members attend a luncheon USFA is hosting for its state partner organization. Erin contends only a few staff members need to go and others could stay at the office to complete their work. She worries it is inefficient to send them all while also trying to keep project activities on schedule. Ranny disagrees, firmly stating, "No, I told them they could all go. USFA needs to provide for its staff, so they stay happy." Enabled by U.S. support for their leadership, Cambodian managers at USFA were able to challenge American ideas and offer new ones to American managers on the topic of staff compensation.

Ranny uses the imaginaries of both Asia and the West to her advantage. She attributes to Western donors that she was able to become a strong female leader who decides what is best for her staff. She gains power within USFA because USAID wants to empower female leaders. Yet Ranny also draws on the development imaginary of Asia to explain that compensation practices need to make sense within the meaning system of patronage. Due to this, staff describe Ranny herself as a hybrid of Asian and Western development imaginaries. Sokmy explains that Ranny is a product of the Western push for women's leadership in INGOs. But Ranny also takes up the role of a good Asian leader who "takes care" of everyone beneath her. In doing so, she provides a counterpoint to stereotypes in Cambodia that assume only men are successful patrons.

In consequence, the U.S. practices around reporting and compensation are modified and reframed by Cambodian managers to meet staff expectations. At USFA, Cambodian managers have some control over how a portion of the budget is allocated. Managers also push blame for reporting practices onto distant Western others. Finally, American and Cambodian managers ensure that worker compensation is perceived as USFA caring for them. Due to this, staff interpret USFA, and particularly Ranny, as a "good patron" who "takes care of workers."

Here we again see USFA's Cambodian staff succeed in challenging American managers through a hybridization of the Asian and Western development imaginaries. Interestingly, through relational work, Cambodian managers succeed in making USAID's impersonal, transparent budgeting model fit into personalized, patronage financial exchange relationships in Cambodia. Due to this, compared to Japan Services Asia, workers at USFA are much more likely to tell me that USFA is a good place to work, perceiving their employer as a worthy exchange partner.

Imaginaries Reversed

This chapter provides an unexpected finding where USFA's practices are justified through the Asian imaginary, while JSA's fail to be. Here, we see the flexibility of the development imaginaries on full display. In previous chapters, the regional rhetoric of Asian similarity was successfully used to reinforce many of JSA's practices. However, in the case of compensation at JSA, we see it fall flat. This is surprising given the widespread assumption that many Asian countries have similar business and financial practices, which differ from those of the West (Kim 2017). Yet, at JSA, Japanese managers are constrained by private, opaque budgeting practices and a limited budget for staff capacity-building. Financial practices also create a culture of mistrust between employees and Japanese managers when it comes to reporting.

In response to JSA's practices, Cambodian managers parse out differences between Asian nations, labeling Japan as rich and out of touch in comparison to other Asian countries. Additionally, gender trumps Asian similarity as Japanese female leaders are labeled as suspicious patrons. This means that at JSA workers are dissatisfied with the benefits provided. These findings illustrate another unintended outcome of donor gender regimes. Japan's labor market legacy of hiring men in leadership positions ends up impacting Cambodian managers' perception of and interactions with the largely female Japanese leaders.

In contrast, at USFA, Cambodian managers successfully help American managers engage in relational work by undertaking a hybrid use of the development imaginaries. They argue that reporting practices are an annoying Western import, placing blame on distant others. Then they use the capacity-building budget to provide culturally appropriate extras and frame INGO opportunities as gifts to staff. Central to this hybrid model is USFA's Cambodian director, Ranny. She is seen as a product of the West because she is female and the director. Yet she is framed by staff as understanding Asian compensation practices, taking care of her employees. Staff legitimize Ranny's authority, perceiving her as a successful broker between the Asian and Western imaginaries. In this case, through hybrid use of the imaginaries, USFA is successful in providing "Asian-style" compensation and is seen as a "good patron" by employees.

These findings point out just how useful it could be to examine relational work, patronage, and expectations about employee-employer relationships in transnational workplaces in the Global South. Workers in nations across the Global South frequently make sense of money through the lens of patronage (Smith 2003). Yet patronage is often written off by donors and scholars alike as a corrupt political system or something to defend organizational budgets against, instead of also being taken seriously as a cultural schema that provides understandings about money in social relationships. At USFA, despite transparent budgeting's original purpose of combating some patronage practices, Cambodian managers' ability to adapt it through relational work means employees are satisfied with their employer. To improve accounting or compensation practices in INGOs or other transnational work settings, it is not possible to simply combat (questionable) patronage activities with stricter budgeting mechanisms. Instead, acknowledging that workers interpret finances through the lens of patronage could better inform transnational budgeting and compensation practices.

Here we see the power of actors in the Global South to strategically use the competing development imaginaries to contest and modify incoming financial practices, sometimes in counterintuitive ways. These findings further demonstrate the mutability of development imaginaries. In the next chapter, we will investigate how the use of development imaginaries impacts the ways Cambodian practitioners understand themselves.

Imaginaries and Identities

Modern Development Practitioners in the Global Order

On a warm November day, I stop for lunch with Japan Services Asia (JSA) manager Samnang. As we share *somlaw m-reha* (Cambodian bitter melon soup) and *dri broma bong dio* (an omelet with dried fish), I ask him about his future career goals. Samnang explains that in his current job, he befriends officials and "shows them how following the way of Japan could help Cambodia." He goes on to tell me, after working at JSA, it is his dream to get a job in Phnom Penh at the Ministry of Health or the Public Health Division of the Ministry of Education. He believes that "a strong government will help his nation develop" and he wants to be part of it. A year later, Samnang informs me he has successfully moved into a health education job within the Ministry of Education.

During my time at U.S. Family Aid (USFA), I go to lunch with the staff member I share my cubicle with, Chantrea. As we share *cha drap psych chrue* (fried eggplant with pork dish) and fried rice, I ask Chantrea a similar question about her future career ambitions. Chantrea reports she has worked for four different INGOs in her career: a local NGO, one funded by Australia's bilateral agency, another by the UK's bilateral agency, and now she works for USFA, funded by USAID. Each previous job has ended when the donor's project concludes. She reports that she enjoys working in development and research. "I want our city to be like Bangkok . . . where donors and INGOs can put regional headquarters, host conferences, and give NGO workers permanent jobs." Her career goal is to land a permanent position in a development organization. About three months after I meet her, Chantrea lands her dream job and leaves USFA to work in a permanent position at the United Nations' Development Programme office in Phnom Penh.

The career trajectories of the two practitioners above introduce the differences in what workers at JSA and USFA understand to be the ideal career trajectory of a modern development professional. In the process of implementing aid projects, Cambodian practitioners use the development imaginaries to construct distinctive identities and career aspirations. The gender regimes and professional identities coming from Tokyo and Washington, D.C., influence, but do not dictate, the identities Cambodian workers create. Instead, Cambodian practitioners engage the imaginaries of Asia and the West to create differing career ambitions than what donors might immediately envision for them. In constructing these new identities, practitioner beliefs about class, race, gender, and Cambodia's national advancement as well as the role of development workers in that advancement come to the forefront.

Transnational Careers and Identity Work

In capitalist societies, people's identities and self-worth are deeply tied to their work and career aspirations (Mount 2024). For example, in most countries, gender norms tell men they must be successful breadwinners to be "real" men (Matlon 2022). This makes work particularly essential to men's self-perception and self-esteem. The social environment of transnational workplaces, including INGOs, are contact zones where workers encounter new incoming beliefs and opportunities for reconsidering their identities and career trajectories. At the same time, incoming beliefs are translated into a recipient nation's cultural context and workers' existing self-perceptions. As identity work commonly involves crafting the self in relation to or opposition to an "other," in making sense of transnational work experiences, workers frequently express career aspirations through the lens of class, gender, race, and national identities (Alexander 2006; Balogun 2020; Matlon 2022; Mount 2024; Radhakrishnan 2011).

For instance, Radhakrishnan (2011) studied Indian women who work in foreign-owned information technology (IT) firms. By taking IT jobs, middle-class Indian women challenged traditional ideas about womanhood in India by working outside of the home, constructing new middle-class, professional identities. Yet these women also make sense of their new identities by contrasting "good" Indian families to the "falling apart" families of the West where divorce rates are high. They do so to craft an identity that hybridizes international ideas about professional women alongside "appropriate" Indian femininity and motherhood. Professional Indian women in IT come to symbolize what it means to be a "good" Indian woman to a transnational audience. Here, we see ideas about social class, race, gender, and India's place in the global order intertwine in the creation of new professional identities. Engaging notions of national advancement alongside cultural traditions, like appropriate Indian motherhood, career trajectories become a space to stake a nation's claim in the modern global order while simultaneously uplifting a nation's cultural traditions.

Like these Indian IT workers, Cambodian practitioners try to construct aspirations about what it means to be "modern" and yet maintain cultural traditions. Previous research on aid work often assumes that aid workers encounter "modern" ideas about their identities, such as individualism, economic success, gender equality, and so on from donors in the West. In contrast, a recipient nation's culture was associated with upholding tradition (Fernandes 2017; Roth 2015). Yet workers at JSA and USFA complicate the association between the West as modern and local culture as traditional when they construct notions of what it would mean to be "modern" in a world where the West's model is not the sole path to development. As we will see, notions of what is modern and traditional, alongside beliefs about class, race, gender, and nation, are being employed in complex ways within the development imaginaries to define practitioner career aspirations.

The Limits of the Donor Gender Regime at Japan Services Asia

To summarize previous chapters, at Japan Services Asia (JSA), Japan's donor gender regime assumes the state should provide all women with low-cost, quality maternal health services; women will be the primary caretakers of the family; and it is not appropriate to discuss gender inequalities directly. At JSA, the interpretation of these assumptions through the development imaginary ends up in project activities that support public health workers. Cambodian workers also justify promoting masculine medical authority over women's bodies, the hybridization of traditional and biomedical practices, and a vision of a modern Asia where men are primary breadwinners and mothers take on most of the household and childcare labor.

At JSA, as practitioners implement aid activities, they construct new ways of thinking about themselves and their careers. However, these new identities differ from the identities staff at INGO headquarters and donor organizations in Japan believe they are imparting to INGO workers. Interviewees in Tokyo are highly focused on increasing the capacity of state officials. They do not assume the career trajectories of Cambodian INGO workers will expand beyond the INGO sector. This is due in large part to the social position of INGO workers in Tokyo.

As detailed earlier, the nonprofit and INGO sector in Tokyo is newer and, for this reason, less professionalized than that of Washington, D.C. Due to its late development, the domestic nonprofit as well as the INGO sector in Tokyo remains small and has limited funding compared to Western nations. One INGO interviewee in Tokyo reports many Japanese INGOs are "small so it is more difficult to have the capacity to write the proposal and everything in English. That is why we do not get as much funding from foreign donors outside of Japan."

The small sector is also highly female-dominated. This is because INGOs are not considered high-paying or long-term workplaces, compared to private sector or government jobs. When I ask JSA headquarters staff about their career plans, most women say they will quit after they have kids, or this is a job they got after their children were older. One headquarters staff member explains that although she loves traveling for her job, she plans to quit and become a stay-at-home mom after her son is born. The exception to this was the role of INGO director, which was frequently filled by men. Occasionally, these men were passionate activists, but more frequently they were older, retired businessmen charged with fundraising for the organization through corporate connections. For this reason, in Tokyo, INGO work is perceived as low-paid, feminized, charity work, or a place for retirees.

In consequence, interviewees in Tokyo do not assume that it would be possible for INGO workers (a marginalized, feminized job in Japan) to become state officials (highly sought after, and masculinized positions in Japan). When asked directly about what they believe Cambodian workers' career goals should be, some Tokyo interviewees muse they might become public clinic workers in rural areas or go to work for another INGO. But the idea that practitioners might choose to use their networks to become state officials does not occur to practitioners in Tokyo. Despite this, as we will see, this is exactly what JSA staff do.

"Modern" Development Professionals as State Officials

The modern worker identity constructed at JSA is an implicitly *male* and *Asian* government official who can effectively implement public services. As we saw in chapter 2, male staff at JSA spend an inordinate amount of time building personal relationships with government officials. It is the belief of JSA's Japanese and Cambodian practitioners that personal connections are key for JSA to support government officials in upgrading their capacity to implement public health services. However, these relationships have an unintended consequence. Khmer workers develop new career aspirations to eventually become state officials. As we are driving from Steung Treng to Phnom Penh, I sit in the backseat listening to Boran and Samnang's conversation. Discussing their meeting with the director of the provincial health department, Samnang reports he believes the director will put a good word in for him when he applies for a government position. Boran listens attentively and wonders aloud if he could work in the provincial health department in Taeko where his family of origin is located.

JSA managers reinforce these career ambitions among themselves by reminding each other that donors will eventually go home, and state-building is the "Asian way" of doing development. Samnang encourages Boran to consider applying to work in public health in Taeko since "JSA and JICA's money won't be here forever" and the state is "where these programs will go in the future anyway, that is what we're working for." Samnang goes on to assert that once he gets a ministry position in Phnom Penh, he can help Boran to get one as well.

On a later date, Boran tells me he found working closely with public officials difficult at first. When he was younger, he was nervous about treating officials as his friends. Now he has become much more comfortable. He says he often goes out drinking with officials and they act as if he is their equal. This means he can tell them about what he has seen in Japan, and they can discuss freely how to implement the Cambodian Ministry of Health's policies. He feels this work can make a difference. For Boran, having respected public officials treat him as an equal and listen to his advice is very personally empowering. He explains that as he learned to befriend them like this and earned their respect and friendship, his self-confidence also increased. "I am not just the little guy from a village anymore." Boran's family still lives in Taeko on a farm, but working at JSA for ten years has allowed him to attain middle-class status, travel the country, gain a medical degree, and befriend well-respected state officials. Working for JSA clearly modifies Boran's identity and self-worth.

Even though it was not the intention of Japanese donors to train new state officials, many JSA staff members describe ambitions to work in the public sector in the future. Most managers came to see JSA as a stepping stone for moving into government careers. This illustrates, again, that practitioners choose to highlight some incoming messages from donors and ignore others. Workers draw on the Japanese gender regime's emphasis on a strong state yet, at the same time, go against the career trajectories practitioners in Tokyo envision for them.

For Sovann and Boran, it was not until after working at JSA and making friendships with officials that they began to see government work as a possible career move. Sovann thinks working in the district health department in Kandal (a province just outside Phnom Penh) is an appealing career move because he would no longer need to travel each week. A few staff members wanted to become officials before working at JSA. Before coming to JSA, Samnang, whose father is a high-level government employee, already considered working in a ministry to be his eventual career plan. It was through his own father's connection to JICA officials that he got his current job at JSA. Samnang believes working for JSA before moving into the public sector will build his social network and allow him to see how people really live in rural areas, knowledge that will serve him well as a government official. He also believes that having connections in JICA and the Japanese embassy will assist him.

As discussed in chapter 4, female workers are often in lower-level positions at JSA and work more closely with villagers. For this reason, they do not form the same close relationships with provincial- and national-level government officials. Consequently, a few women workers did aspire to government jobs, but when they did, they were often jobs at the subnational level. Through their work, assistants get to know villagers in JSA's target areas. They call village leaders ahead of time to organize events, gather information from village chiefs, arrange meetings with mothers, and talk warmly with participants and village leaders at JSA community events. Aiding upper-level staff in implementing health trainings, assistants are called lou kru or naek kru (teacher) by mothers and other villagers. One assistant, Chhy, explains that when he hears other villagers, even older villagers, call him teacher, "I feel so good. . . . I do not know if I deserve it . . . but I feel so good when I hear them say this." At JSA, although *who* they build relationships with and status among is different, all staff list relationship-building or the social ties they gain from their job as important to their professional identities.

Some program assistants thought these community connections might afford them access to local government jobs. Sopheap, who had been a program assistant for almost a year, thinks her improved status in the community helped to build her confidence that she could achieve her dream of working as a teacher at the local public school. With midwife training, Chea, another program assistant, thought she might eventually become a midwife at a local public health clinic.

Consequently, at JSA, ideal future career identities as state workers in a "strong Asian state" were justified as the path to Asian development. Workers made this argument by juxtaposing a strong Asian state to Western reliance on civil society and on liberal democracy, which was frequently portrayed as in decline. For instance, Sovann tells me "Cambodia has been dominated by Western donors for so long, since after the Pol Pot times, their experts are always coming here but their way doesn't always work for us. Cambodia is not Europe." Or, as most of my fieldwork took place during the first Trump presidency, Samnang laughs, citing Brexit and "America's funny president," and asks, "Why should Cambodia follow that path?" In this way, JSA staff argue for a new path to development, discounting the West. They believe it is state officials who will play a key role in advancing Cambodian society and envision themselves in this role in the future.

It must be noted that, at JSA, staff buy into the model that "Asian" nations should have developmental states, despite the continued limitations of their own government in reality. While the Cambodian government has made great strides in economic growth and infrastructure, it continues to lag in social services and equitable growth (World Bank 2018). It also goes unmentioned by JSA staff that the Cambodian state is a constrained democracy with a single dominant party that does not necessarily represent its citizens' interests. Thus, deployment of the Asian development imaginary to envision the Cambodian state as a strong developmental state that provides health services may be an unattainable aspiration. Time will tell. Nevertheless, the construction of worker identities at JSA engages specific forms of class consumption as well as beliefs about gender, race, and nation.

Class, Gender, and Race in Identity Formation at Japan Services Asia

For JSA staff, particularly male workers who want higher-level government jobs, the middle-class identity of future state officials is pursued through specific consumption patterns. Around the world, consumption is often an integral part of how people in the Global South fashion what it means to be "modern" in their self-presentations and identities (Matlon 2022; Mojola 2014). Particularly in Cambodia, successful masculinity is now associated with having multiple mobile phones, the ability to use modern technologies like computers and tablets, and wearing East Asian and Western inspired fashions (Jacobsen 2011).

The construction of new identities for transnational workers frequently entails consumption. In Radhakrishnan's (2011) study of Indian IT professionals, she finds that Indian women combine "modern" consumption patterns with a focus on "Indian" family values. Female workers buy modern items that they can justify as being of service to the family, like refrigerators or cars. Here we see them define spending lavishly on the family as part of what it means to be a modern Indian IT worker and mother. At JSA, workers also define consumption patterns that match their modern professional identity.

The purchase of specific middle-class status symbols that are associated with Cambodian state officials is central to the construction of identity for JSA workers that aspire to be government officials. Their relationships with officials afford them knowledge about state officials' consumption patterns. Male staff purchase professional clothing, electronics, and particular types of golden jewelry for themselves. While many of these items are status symbols consumed by the Cambodian middle class more generally, JSA workers carefully bought items preferred by state officials, which were not considered "too Western," or items that exhibited what they referred to as national and/or Asian pride.

For instance, high-level political officials in Cambodia frequently wear large gold and diamond rings and watches. Boran tells me gold jewelry is deeply Cambodian and goes all the way back to Cambodian-Chinese trade in pre-Angkor and Angkor Empire times.[1] He draws on a long history, as gold played an important role in Cambodian upper-class accessories and temple decorations all the way back to the ancient Oc-Èo civilization that existed in the region in the first century B.C. (Jacques 2020). Also, as noted in chapter 3, men are compared to gold and women to cloth in the fourteenth-century traditional Khmer code of conduct for women. This illustrates yet another way gold has played a role in Cambodian cultural traditions and masculinity.

Several of JSA's managers also purchase traditional Cambodian carved wooden furniture, frequently stopping along the road to shop for these pieces on our rides back and forth from Phnom Penh. Due to rampant deforestation, wood for this furniture is in increasingly short supply. This wooden furniture is another status symbol associated with national pride and Cambodian tradition. For male managers, this type of consumption allowed them to display their middle-class status alongside pride in their culture and Asian-ness.

Program assistants also found working for an INGO afforded them newfound consumption options that brought respect from other villagers. Assistants are provided with access to JSA's cars, tablets, and cell phones—symbols of status in rural Steung Treng. Their salaries also allowed them to purchase clothing, purses, and accessories for themselves and other family members. Several assistants believed access to consumer goods like these might help them increase their status and access public jobs in the future.

While it was acceptable for female assistants to dream of taking jobs in rural public schools or health clinics, male managers at JSA made it clear that the career ambition to be a high-ranking state official is available only to men. As Samnang explains, it is important that his wife's job is "secondary" as her main role is to care for their children. Linking this perspective to "traditional" rural Cambodian life, he states "it has always been this way, you see, even in the village, the woman stays back to care for children, the garden, and the animals, while the husband goes out into the fields or forest." Samnang believes that men in Asia have historically left the home for work, and this makes men better suited for public-facing government leadership roles.

Similarly, pointing to Japan, Boran explains that women frequently prioritize staying home with their children. He lists headquarters staff members from Tokyo he has interacted with who later became stay-at-home moms. For male staff at JSA, as the economy develops in Cambodia, men will be increasingly enabled to keep their wives at home or, at most, run informal businesses at home that can be easily combined with childcare. He believes, like other male staff members at JSA, that it is men who will be in the driver's seat of Cambodia's advancement in the public sector.

The gendering of JSA's career aspirations is clear in the way women's ambitions to work in the government sector are treated by male staff. Chea, who has midwife training, could have been introduced to public health workers by male staff to help her on her way to becoming a midwife at a public clinic. Instead, they told Chea that eventually she would marry and settle down, so there was no point in introducing her to clinic doctors. Such practices reinforced the idea that the ideal state official was implicitly male.

Finally, the Asian development imaginary enables JSA staff to envision a new international order that challenges the historic global racial hierarchy. Out in the field one day, Samnang and I encounter World Vision volunteers who are organizing villagers to build a well. He explains to me that Cambodia no longer needed "white Christians" to build wells and hospitals. In the near future, the Cambodian state would be better able to take care of its citizens with the help of Asian donors. In another example, one day I attend a short planning meeting between Samnang and Dr. Mao. Dr. Mao tells Samnang he is working with KOICA and expresses how impressed he is with Korea's economic advancement. He thinks the West has less money than it once did. They both agree that they hope in the future, "those with the money will be Asian." This use of the competing imaginaries empowers staff to challenge the traditional global racial and economic hierarchy that has been in place since European colonization (Noor 2021).

Yet, male staff also intertwine rhetoric about class and colorism to police the boundaries around the coveted role of state health official. One day, after explaining the chain of command to two newly hired staff members, Sovann goes on to joke to Boran that "the chain of command can be seen in skin tone. It is clear who will move up into state jobs from here." Although all program staff are Khmer, program assistants are hired out of rural Steung Treng. Growing up in Steung Treng, assistants often help their families with farm work, so their skin is noticeably darker in complexion due to sun exposure, a sign of class status in Cambodia. Program assistants, who are largely female, are associated with "rural tradition" and lower on the social hierarchy compared to upper-level expert male staff who have only held professional jobs and live middle-class lives in Phnom Penh, coming to Steung Treng each week for work. However, this rhetoric that associates program assistants with rural tradition in order to demean them is employed by the same managers who valorized rural traditions in gender relations to reject the workplace equality of the "modern West" above. This illustrates that, at JSA, Khmer managers engage simultaneously in contradictory rhetoric about class, gender, and race.

JSA workers envision a "modern" development worker that is inherently a male government official working within the "Asian" model of state-led development. This identity is in line with research that finds men in Southeast Asia are increasingly constructing identities that contest dominant Western forms of masculinity (Hoang 2013). The construction of JSA's worker identity challenges existing global power relations. In envisioning state officials as key players in Cambodia's advancement, it defies long dominant notions of neoliberal economic development that disinvests in the state. JSA workers create an alternative "Asian" path to development alongside their new career trajectories. Yet, while it challenges some hierarchies, the construction of JSA's professional identity reinforces others. Male staff use the Asian imaginary and conflicting notions of tradition to simultaneously contest racialized global inequalities while upholding oppressive hierarchies based on class, skin color, and gender in their own nation and region.

The Contradictions of the Gender Regime at U.S. Family Aid

As the previous chapters have illustrated, at USFA, the U.S. gender regime fosters support for the private and nonprofit healthcare sector. It values women's economic empowerment and consumer choice in maternal and reproductive healthcare. It also fosters a professionalized work environment where men and women are technically equal, yet it leaves women to cope with the requirements of motherhood on their own. At USFA, the interpretation of the donor gender regime through the development imaginaries creates project activities that support the development of the nonprofit sector and private clinics. Cambodian practitioners also hybridize notions of Western gender equality and Asian family to modify USFA's aid programming and workplace practices.

Like JSA staff, as Cambodian practitioners at USFA implement development activities, they construct new professional identities and career trajectories. However, again, these new identities do not flow neatly from the directives of Washington, D.C. Interviewees in Washington, D.C., present a contradictory picture of what they believe INGO worker career trajectories in recipient nations will be. These ideas flow from the U.S.'s own history of nonprofits and INGOs discussed in chapter 5. The U.S. has a very long history of nonprofit organizing and highly professionalized nonprofit and INGO sectors. The U.S. government relies heavily on INGOs to help dispense foreign aid (or at least it did before the 2025 USAID shutdown that will be discussed in the next chapter). Due to the country's long nonprofit history, the sectors are highly funded, influential, and professionalized in comparison to Japan's.

Existing in this context, interviewees in Washington, D.C., have mixed responses when it comes to the ideal career trajectories of INGO workers in the Global South. Some believe INGOs provide stopgap social services and in an ideal world they will no longer be needed. Eventually, those services will be provided by the state or market. One interviewee explains "it's ideal that INGOs work themselves out of the job." Some INGO interviewees in Washington, D.C., believed that future practitioners in the Global South would need to find jobs in the private sector or INGOs would become private firms themselves.

One interviewee in Washington, D.C., explains that funding is decreasing to NGOs globally. In response to decreased resources, he has seen several successful cases of INGOs becoming research or consulting firms, marketing their skills to the private sector. He describes an example of a women's NGO that provides sexual harassment prevention trainings to businesses. He has also encountered an agricultural NGO that provides workshops on efficient farming practices for private agriculture companies. He goes on to say, "I've even heard of NGOs that conduct internal evaluations of businesses to assess whether their Corporate Social Responsibility funds are addressing the Sustainable Development Goals." In a similar vein, several interviewees thought NGOs should become social enterprises, doing things like setting up a hotel or restaurant business. Then they would use the profits of that business to support their social service work.

Alternatively, working in Washington, D.C.'s highly professionalized INGO sector, other interviewees thought INGOs in the Global South might have a future that would look similar to the nonprofit sector in the U.S. In this future, INGO country offices would be localized and then seek funding from their own government. Local NGOs would eventually develop their own vibrant, professionalized domestic nonprofit sectors. One Washington, D.C., donor interviewee explains, "the hope is eventually their governments start funding NGOs." Working within these two visions, workers at USFA's home office construct their vision of a "modern" development professional who is a cosmopolitan, middle-class global citizen, and an expert in the development field.

"Modern" Development Professionals as Cosmopolitan Experts

Cambodian practitioners at USFA encounter the two above visions from Washington, D.C. In response to the first one, USFA practitioners tell me there are not enough jobs in the private sector, and they scoff at the idea that every NGO worker in Phnom Penh could move into a private sector job. Additionally, to the idea that NGOs should be run as consulting firms or social enterprises, Cambodian practitioners think this has some, but only limited, feasibility. They report there are currently many NGOs in Phnom Penh attempting the private firm model due to decreased donor funding, so the market of NGO consultants is already flooded. Additionally, NGO social enterprises in Cambodia rarely make enough money to go entirely without donor support, particularly since tourism declined post-COVID-19. In consequence, USFA practitioners do not find the idea that eventually most INGOs and practitioners will become part of the private sector feasible.

USFA practitioners do partially enact the second future career trajectory vision coming from the U.S. They agree with the need to build up the INGO sector in Cambodia. But, in Washington, D.C., American practitioners assume that, in this model, INGOs will eventually be localized. This would mean donor funding is just a temporary measure, and the Cambodian state will eventually fund its nonprofit sector. Khmer practitioners ignore such comments when they envision a growing professionalized development sector in Phnom Penh. They do not believe that the Cambodian government or private sector will ever fund a large number of NGOs or nonprofits. This is not unreasonable given the Cambodian government's legal restrictions on INGOs.

Instead, Cambodian practitioners envision a future where development donors continue providing most of the funding to INGOs, although they believe the makeup of donor nations may change. They describe a future in which Phnom Penh could be a hub of international development in Southeast Asia, similar to Bangkok. USFA practitioners frequently reference Bangkok, a development hub where many INGO regional headquarters are located, as the path Cambodia should take.

Within this future for Cambodia's development sector, practitioners express a desire to move up to bilateral or multilateral agencies that pay more and offer permanent positions. Darika started her career at a local NGO, moved to a smaller private development research firm, and then moved to her current role in budget and contracts at USFA. She explains to me that she wants to keep gaining skills at USFA that will eventually allow her to move up into a bilateral agency, like USAID, DFAT (the Australian bilateral agency), or KOICA (the Korean bilateral agency). Other staff members express ambitions to become INGO directors, like USFA's director, Ranny.

Practitioners at USFA are just as aware of changing international power dynamics as JSA's staff. Considering their future, USFA workers frequently hybridize narratives about Asia and the West, arguing for a future of "partnership." By partnership they mean there would be more equal cooperation between Asian nations, including Cambodia, and Western ones. Cambodian practitioners imagine that, in the future, nations in Southeast Asia, like Thailand and Singapore, will become more important aid donors in the region. Imagining their own role in the path Cambodia should take to advancement, USFA workers envision that, in the future, Southeast Asian practitioners will have more power in determining the types of development projects funded in their region. One practitioner explains that as Southeast Asian nations grow in economic power, there will be more reason for donors to listen to us, other Southeast Asian nations will become donors, and we will be here to tell them what Cambodia needs when that happens.

Consequently, USFA workers push back on Western dominance in the development sector less directly than staff at JSA. Nevertheless, they still envision a future where Cambodians are considered the expert development professionals within Southeast Asia, cooperating on increasingly equal footing with donors. The construction of this ideal professional identity at USFA also engages classed, raced, and gendered identities.

Class, Gender, and Race in Identity Formation at U.S. Family Aid

Key to this expert development professional identity is middle-class status.[2] Over lunch, Darika tells me that her mother and father sell goods in an open-air market on the outskirts of the capital city. Her parents worked hard for her to go to college in Phnom Penh and are very proud she has an office job, dresses professionally, does not work outside in the heat, and eventually will help take care of them. All married staff members at USFA, male or female, are in couples where both partners work, a necessity to maintain their middle-class lifestyles. Spouses have a variety of middle-class jobs such as banker, doctor, development professional, hotel manager, tailor, restaurant owner, with one government official.

When it comes to the consumption markers of their professional identity, USFA workers pursue what I call "Pan-Asian" cosmopolitan respectability, which is different from the consumption pattern we see at JSA (Hoang 2015). Employment at USFA permits staff to work in an office, dress in professional clothing, and maintain a five-day work week, all important markers of a middle-class and "modern" lifestyle in Cambodia. Status symbols, while important to all USFA practitioners, are consumed in gendered ways. After saving up, male workers purchase status symbols such as phones, cars, or watches. When monitoring and evaluation specialist Panh gets a new smart watch, several colleagues stop him to inquire about it. Men often admire and purchase high-tech electronics from China, Japan, and South Korea.

Similarly, women save up for and complement each other often on new designer-brand purses or outfits. USFA staff, particularly women, say they imitate South Koreans in their pursuit of a middle-class aesthetic and lifestyle. Like many other Southeast Asia nations, South Korean popular culture, including drama, movies, and music, has fully inundated Cambodia, particularly in urban areas. The South Korean aesthetic is admired by citizens all over Southeast Asia, and Cambodia is no exception (Hoang 2015). Staff frequently get haircuts, makeup, clothing, and accessories to pursue this aesthetic. One colleague explains to me that she hopes that by using Korean skincare, maybe she can look as light and beautiful as the women in the K-dramas. She thinks many Cambodian women are inspired by the Koreans, how fast they could develop their country, and how beautiful they look.

In another instance, Chantrea comments on the fact that Thailand and Vietnam are doing better economically than Cambodia. Drawing on colorism to define Pan-Asian cosmopolitan respectability, she brings my attention to the fact that citizens of Thailand and Vietnam often have lighter skin tones, in comparison to Cambodia, Laos, or Myanmar. These examples all draw on the racial hierarchy within Asia, noting the lighter skin of many Korean, Thai, and Vietnamese citizens. Most female practitioners at USFA believe skin-lightening products are important for a middle-class lifestyle. Again, we see the desire to differentiate oneself from "poorer" Asians in both rural areas and less developed countries. At USFA, racial and class hierarchy are less explicit than at JSA, where male staff literally pointed out the differentiations in office positions by skin tone. But the need for a lighter skin tone is still intertwined with the middle-class status USFA workers pursue. These beliefs are held despite the economic and democratic successes of nations like India, where people frequently have a darker skin tone than South Korean or Vietnamese people. USFA practitioners make sense of the racial and economic order of Asia through a hierarchy of skin tone, with lighter-skinned Asians being at the top.

Additionally, middle-class workers valued the ability to send their children to expensive after-school education programs in Phnom Penh, which are popular throughout East Asia. At lunch one day, USFA staff member Chantrea tells me it is important to her to maintain a middle-class lifestyle through INGO work so her kids, who go to private school and after-school lessons to learn Chinese, can do even better than her. When I ask why Chinese over English, she explains that she has two reasons. She can teach them English, and she thinks Chinese might be the future language for work and business in Cambodia. Chantrea is aware that, although she works at a Western-style development organization, in the future her children will need to know Chinese. Her decision illustrates that even practitioners at a Western-funded INGO believe in an Asian future. Cambodian workers at USFA have a vision of Cambodia's future where Asia and the West are on more equal footing. They teach their children Chinese and pursue a South Korean aesthetic.

Another status symbol that upholds cosmopolitan respectability, which I did not see often at JSA, was a love for international travel. As discussed in chapter 5, JSA only enables upper-level staff to travel to Japan after working at JSA for over five years. In contrast, USFA offers more frequent opportunities for travel to conferences and workshops both domestically and abroad. USFA workers are excited about the opportunity for travel afforded by their jobs. As Sophy says, "This job allows me to be a jetsetter." Staff often post photos of themselves at international conferences around the world on social media. She describes the opportunity to travel the world as well as the chance to meet and go out with new female friends as the best parts of working for Western INGOs.

Sophy is not alone. Most practitioners at USFA really appreciate the ability to go out to eat and drink with their coworkers outside of work. Srey-na explains that it is amazing to work at INGOs from the West because one can make like-minded female friends, go out to exciting new restaurants and bars in Phnom Penh, and be acknowledged as someone who works in the international development community. I frequently accompanied USFA staff to restaurants serving international foods or high-end bars. While JSA program managers are also middle-class Phnom Penh residents, due to their distinctive consumption style, they did not express the same meaningful connection with going out to international bars and restaurants in the expatriate neighborhoods of Phnom Penh. This activity was tied to an identity of Pan-Asian cosmopolitan respectability and development expertise pursued by USFA staff.

Committed to middle-class lifestyles, USFA employees worry about the insecurity entailed in INGO work. As Chantrea's story introducing this chapter shows, USFA workers were often employed previously on several short-term grants at different INGOs. Typically, after getting a large bilateral or multilateral grant, INGOs hire new workers. But, after the completion of that grant, many of those new workers are laid off. For instance, the monitoring and evaluation specialist at USFA, Panh, previously worked on USAID projects at three other INGOs. At USFA, 60 percent of the USAID project staff had been hired on just for that project.

Staff lucky enough to have worked at USFA for more than five years were often shuffled from one grant to another. A member of the program team, Sophal, informs me that he previously worked on malaria and family planning projects at USFA, until those grants ended. Then he was switched to the new USAID project. However, he still worries that if USFA does not get another big grant, he may have to take a break or look for a new place to work. He tells me that practitioners need to be flexible and jump on opportunities to succeed in this field. But, he tells me, the good news is that Western donors are all so similar that practitioners can easily move from one to another.

This funding situation causes USFA staff to be constantly on the lookout for their next jobs. INGO staff, who often meet one another at conferences and workshops, share information with one another about upcoming big grants and which INGOs might win them. Such connections assist practitioners in finding the next INGO opportunity when one grant ends. While practitioners might be middle class, this status is precarious as most USFA practitioners express that their families absolutely could not maintain their current lifestyle without their income.

Despite this insecurity, most USFA staff envision career advancement within the international development sector. It is not completely unheard of for U.S.-based INGO workers to move into government careers, particularly in the early 2000s, when there were a limited number of skilled workers in Cambodia. However, with the current geopolitical relations between the U.S. and Cambodia, no USFA worker expressed a desire to move into government work in the future. One worker wanted to start her own clothing store, and another was considering moving into microfinance. All other USFA staff saw their future in the development sector.

Finally, working at USFA, staff encounter trainings and workshops that ask them to critically consider gender. When I arrive at USFA, the director introduces me, letting everyone know I am doing a research project on NGOs, health, and gender. Staff nod in familiarity. Yet, as we saw in previous chapters, staff also face difficulties integrating gender rhetoric into the Cambodian context. One day, USFA worker Sreynich is translating a document. She informs me the real problem is that "gender" cannot be translated easily into Khmer. She tells me she appreciates how much she has learned from the gender workshops of Western donors. The workshops changed the way she thinks about herself, her work, and her family. But, she explains, "when we just use the English word, gender, everyone assumes it is coming from the West. So, we must find ways to talk about these issues . . . more indirectly."

Exposure to incoming gendered beliefs and the need to translate them into the Cambodian context has varying impacts on USFA practitioner identities. When I explain my comparative research project, USFA staff have a lot to say about Asian and Western donors and gender. A few staff members purport that "the culture of Japan or South Korea is closer," "Japanese NGOs must better understand how to work with Khmer families," "Japan does not intervene in culture, like the West, but helps women become healthier mothers." In this rhetoric is the assumption that in following the path of other Asian nations, development can be achieved without sacrificing "traditional" or "Asian" values, such as family loyalty.

USFA's monitoring and evaluation expert, Panh, informed me that "culture could not change" and "gender is pushed on us from the U.S. but it is not the Cambodian way." He engages with the language of gender equality solely to please USAID and other donors from the West. Not unlike male JSA staff, he says that in his household, women take up most of the household labor, and that is how things have always been done in Cambodia.

In stark contrast, other practitioners at USFA express that they are deeply committed to speaking out against gender inequalities. They worry that challenging unequal gender norms will become more difficult with the rise of Asian donors. These practitioners contend that "Western donors have given us tools to think about gender, reproductive health, and how to improve women's lives," but "Asian donors do not talk about gender like the West."

At the same time, several USFA workers push back on the blanket assumption that Asian gender norms are inherently more conservative. USFA's communications manager, Srey-na, considers herself a feminist. She contends that INGO projects must challenge household gender roles to improve women's access to reproductive choices. Srey-na carefully navigates critiques from colleagues that such beliefs are a Western importation. Srey-na claims "we can be Khmer and challenge the idea that women have to do all the cooking, cleaning, and childcare!" She frequently argues that most Cambodian women have historically worked for an income, so this is also part of Cambodian tradition. For Srey-na, these beliefs give her the confidence to say that she is a feminist and speak back to her father and brother. Srey-na says she even feels brave enough to consider going abroad to graduate school in Australia.

But Srey-na and Panh are extreme cases on each end of the gendered beliefs spectrum, with the majority of USFA staff finding a middle ground between what they understand to be Western and Asian gendered beliefs. USFA's director, Ranny, worked on numerous activities encouraging gender equality in her previous jobs at a women's empowerment INGO and then at a bilateral agency. Ranny explains the need for Cambodia to find a way to attain gender equality within Khmer and Asian traditions. She proudly tells me about a time, at her previous job at a women's empowerment INGO, when she had to go up against the owners of Heineken. Heineken owns a well-known beer brand in Southeast Asia, Tiger Beer. At that time, Tiger Beer required female distributors known as "beer girls" that work at many popular restaurants around Phnom Penh to wear only very small skirts and bras to work.

The INGO sent Ranny as a spokesperson to the Heineken corporate meeting. Ranny describes being terrified as she went up to the Heineken board, filled with white men in suits, to give her presentation. She thanked them for providing job opportunities to women but explained that the required outfits are not culturally appropriate for Khmer women; while to a Westerner this requirement might seem like it is empowering women's sexuality, in Cambodia it is not. Ranny told the board that beer girls are harassed and equated with sex workers. She argued that beer girls need to be given a full dress (notably, Tiger's beer girls now do wear full dresses, although they are still quite short by Cambodian standards). Ranny adeptly combined "Western" understandings of female empowerment in the work-force with a narrative about "Asian" understandings of cultural appropri-ateness and gender.

In her own life, Ranny tells me that working for a women's empower-ment organization changed what she thought would be possible for her. She chose to never marry or have children, despite family pressures. Instead, she focused on advancing her career, eventually becoming the director of a large health INGO, USFA. This is a feat she is not sure she could have pulled off without what she learned about gender equality in her job at the women's empowerment NGO.

Yet, it is not only Western gender rhetoric that creates changes in work-er's identities. Another part of the hybridization process is the use of notions of "Asian family" to push back on what staff considered Western individ-ualistic or atomistic notions about society. Staff point out that Asian peo-ples more frequently live with extended families, help each other out with children, and are more deeply embedded in communities. One program manager, Sotheary, expresses shock and sadness Americans must pay people to assist in childcare because they lack the support of extended family. Such rhetoric pushes back on the notion that women in Western nations auto-matically experience more freedoms. In her own life, Sotheary says consid-ering Western gendered beliefs has enabled her to move up at work. But, at the same time, she is committed to serving her extended family and community, which she finds deeply meaningful.

After work, I accompanied Chantrea, Srey-na, and Darika for drinks at a bar and restaurant next door to USFA. We meet up with their friends who work for a few other INGOs and United Nations organizations in Phnom Penh. The women tell stories about their husbands, trade rumors about a few coworkers, and discuss beauty and weight loss. Then, Darika confides in the other two women that she worked hard to follow Srey-na's feminist advice and strike a bargain with her husband. As the women had discussed previously, she told him that she would take care of dinner and the kids six days a week but one day a week, she would go out with the girls. It was only fair that she got some time off. The women giggle and cheer her success and the night off she was currently enjoying. But, at the same time, Darika notes she does not want to lose her connection with her in-laws or be without family support like many Western women. In this case, again,

USFA practitioners aim to strike a balance. In their balance, taking on "too much" from Western gendered beliefs is portrayed as disembedding women from their families.

This hybridization of gendered beliefs is in line with other scholars that find Cambodian women practice "hide and seek resistance" or strategic hybridization of gender norms (Lilja 2017). Cambodian practitioners argue there are many reasons for hybridizing gendered beliefs, including that it is pragmatic, it is difficult for Cambodians to speak directly about gender without facing pushback, and, for those critical of these hybridizations, it is "taking the easy way out" by avoiding hard conversations. Whatever their reasons, USFA's ideal cosmopolitan development experts combine Asian and Western gendered identities in their work and private lives.

Development Professional Identities in Modern Asia

The past three chapters have focused on internal organizational interactions at JSA and USFA. However, I will conclude this chapter on professional identities with one final exemplary story about the director of USFA's sub-grantee organization, Cambodian Development Society (CDS), and his professional identity. One day, having just arrived for fieldwork in Kampong Speu, I have dinner with Rith, the founder and, at that time, director of CDS. Rith tells me about himself, interweaving his personal history with the story of his NGO. He was born in the late 1970s to a farming family in Kampong Speu, at the end of the violent Khmer Rouge regime. As a young person, he lived through enormous political change, including ongoing civil war until 1991 and, shortly thereafter, the arrival of the United Nation's Transitional Authority, which came to assist with the formation of democratic government in Cambodia. Rith describes his family "getting by in whatever way they could" for many years. He also recollects the great hope many Cambodian families had for the future of their country in the early 1990s.

In addition to the construction of a democratic government in Cambodia, the 1980s and 1990s saw the reopening of religious institutions which had been dismantled by the Khmer Rouge. In his teens, Rith decided to become a monk, a way of bringing great merit to his family. As a monk, he learned Buddhist principles as well as how to read and write in English. Yet, by the late 1990s, Rith started noticing the influx of foreign aid funding and proliferation of NGOs in Cambodia. Rith was committed to helping his community and uplifting those in poverty. At the time, he decided one of the best ways to improve the status of his rural community would be to open a vocational and English school for impoverished children. After visiting a number of successful local NGOs, he decided to leave the monkhood to start his local NGO, CDS.[3]

In 2000, CDS began as a small English school and shelter for children, which Rith ran with the help of volunteer monks. Rith was tenacious as an NGO director, traveling to Phnom Penh and Bangkok to network with international donors. He turned out to be a savvy fundraiser and, by the late 2010s, CDS had a budget of almost one million U.S. dollars, to implement education, health, and microfinance projects. Rith recruited donors for his organization, including international NGOs, universities, companies, individuals, and bilateral development agencies from the U.S., Europe, and Australia. Rith explains, "I wanted to help to improve my community, my family, and my country and . . . at that time, starting an NGO was the way to do it."

Prospering as an NGO director, Rith's family is now well off by Kampong Speu's standards. He displays upper middle-class status symbols, such as driving a car and wearing a nice suit, a far cry from the orange monk's robes in which he began his career. With the help of his Scandinavian donors, Rith decided to explore the possibility of creating a "social enterprise"—a business with a social objective. He opened a hotel and yoga retreat, which supports CDS by generating revenue from tourists. It also provides job opportunities for graduates of CDS's vocational school. As director, Rith runs CDS as well as the social enterprise, while always continuing to be on the lookout for the next funding opportunity.

However, during our dinner in May 2019, Rith tells me he thinks "it might be time to change paths" because NGO funding is "not like it was ten years ago." As discussed in the introduction, in 2016, Cambodia was reclassified from a low-income nation to a lower-middle-income nation by the World Bank. Since then, NGO funding from Western donors has declined. Rith believes that to continue to help his family, his community, and his country develop, "a new strategy" is needed. He is considering starting a business.

Before starting the yoga retreat, Rith received support from his donors to attend trainings in management and business networking events in the capital, Phnom Penh. At these forums, Rith had the opportunity to create networks with businessmen from China, Japan, and South Korea, which he believes will be useful in his new commercial venture. He reports to me that it is time for him to "turn to Asian money" where "business and development go together." In 2021, Rith succeeded in his plan. CDS's deputy director is now in charge of the NGO because Rith is the co-CEO of his own company, with a Chinese businessman as his partner. Using his networking skills yet again, Rith and his partner started a construction and sourcing company. The company takes advantage of the numerous infrastructure development loans China, Japan, and South Korea provide to Cambodia.

As Cambodia and its development context changed, so did Rith's trajectory. When religious institutions were reopening and providing aid to rural Cambodians, he became a Buddhist monk. Next, when foreign aid was on the rise and seemed to be Cambodia's most prominent path to development, he became an NGO director. And now, Rith has switched again, to become the CEO of a company which profits from East Asian infrastructure development loans. While he is the only practitioner that I know of who went so far as to start a company, Rith's story is an extreme case of what this chapter has argued. Articulating their identities under conditions of global uncertainty, Cambodians strategically negotiate donor differences as well as economic and geopolitical transformation within their own career aspirations.

The international order shapes how people understand themselves, other people, and their nation. For example, during colonization, a colonizing nation's perceptions were imported to the countries it colonized, becoming part of how colonized peoples perceived themselves (Said 1978). Illustrating this legacy, to this day in Southeast Asia, the media still portray rural people as backwards, traditional, exotic, and inferior—frequently equating them with animals like monkeys. Rural people are juxtaposed to "modern," rational actors in urban areas. Such stereotypes have their roots in colonization (Noor 2021). While colonial histories still shape self-understandings in many nations in Southeast Asia, and the Global South more generally, this chapter has provided insights into how current geographic power transformations are shaping the self-understandings available in new ways.

The increasing economic and geopolitical power of many Asian nations is providing an opportunity for citizens in Southeast Asia to rethink their self-understandings in a new global order (Hoang, Cobb, and Lei 2017). We see this when the development imaginaries are used by practitioners to construct new professional identities in each INGO. These identities are embedded in practitioners' beliefs about the best paths to development for Cambodia, pushing back on the historically dominant belief that the West's path is the sole model. At JSA, practitioners aspire to join a strong Asian state that will play a lead role in Cambodia's advancement and take part in Asia's regional rise. Such an identity is only available to JSA's managers because East Asian developmental states provided an alternative model to the West's neoliberal development. In contrast, USFA staff foresee that Asian donors will increase in power, challenging Western dominance in the development sector. Their career aspiration then is to become Pan-Asian, cosmopolitan development experts who will be needed in a thriving INGO sector with diverse donors.

For practitioners in both INGOs, class, race, and gender are inextricably intertwined in the construction of these new professional identities. While practitioners challenge the global hierarchy in the construction of new identities that contend the time of white, Western dominance over development knowledge is over, they uphold other race and class hierarchies at the same time. Specifically, they reinforce the backwardness of "traditional" rural and economically impoverished identities in Southeast Asia. This is done through domestic colorism in the case of JSA and colorism between Asian nations at USFA. This illustrates that complex, contradictory constructions of race can be used to create universalizing identities, homogenizing all Asians to contest the dominance of the West. Yet, at the same time, practitioners call out specific skin tones, keeping a color hierarchy in place to gatekeep access to new professional identities. Unfortunately, this practice means modern development worker identities are available to largely middle-class practitioners to the exclusion of rural Cambodians. This demonstrates something feminists have long argued, that "upward mobility and interpreting oneself as an autonomous individual are 'resources' that are distributed unequally" (Mount 2024: 12).

We also see gendered beliefs come into new career aspirations. At JSA, a hierarchy in which men are at the top is reinforced as part of the modern development professional identity of a state official. This is justified through the idea that "traditional" Asian gender norms promote male breadwinners. In contrast, at USFA, practitioners strategically craft identities that combine Asian and Western beliefs. They hybridize gendered ideas they attribute to Asia and the West to carve out a slightly more liberatory space for themselves, such as Darika getting a night off each week from her household and childcare duties. To many USFA practitioners, the "modern" Asian woman preserves Asian values like motherhood and communalism but also advocates for incremental change.

The development imaginaries, alongside complex notions of what is modern and traditional, are employed to remake the self-understandings and envision the new identities for practitioners and their place in Cambodia's path to national advancement. In doing so, practitioners follow Chen's (2010) description of inter-Asian referencing that argues "using Asia as an imaginary anchoring point can allow societies in Asia to become one another's reference points, so that the understanding of the self can be transformed, and subjectivity rebuilt" and, in doing so, nations in the region are creating their own relationship with the concept of Asia itself (xv).

Conclusion

The power behind the culture of U.S. imperialism comes from its ability to insert itself into a geocolonial space as the imaginary figure of modernity, and as such, the natural object of identification from which the local people are to learn.

—KUAN-HSING CHEN, *ASIA AS METHOD*

The central contribution of this book is that it illuminates how aid practitioners in Cambodia are using regional imaginaries of development, and the meanings of gender within them, to shift the world order. As Chen's quote (2010: 177) above demonstrates, since World War II, the dominance of Western development models has been upheld through "the recirculation and rearticulation of myths of (American) origin" (Alexander 2006: 5). In contrast, this book documents the processes through which new myths, or development imaginaries, are circulated as we enter an era where the world has multiple, regional centers of power.

As we have seen, alongside aid programming, foreign donors from the U.S. and Japan bring to Cambodia distinctive understandings about the role the state, market, civil society, and gender should play in development. In response to foreign aid donors and regional changes, development practitioners in Cambodia imagine two model paths to development, one "Asian" and the other "Western." Cambodian practitioners draw on these two imaginaries in debates about their nation's advancement, using them to challenge or modify one another, rather than fully adopting either one wholesale. In doing so, Cambodians construct their own hybrid models that envision the role the state, market, and civil society should play in development, the place of men and women in the workplace and families, and the position of Cambodia, and themselves, in the global order. Consequently, development practitioners in Cambodia are engaging in the microfoundational processes that are creating foreign aid regionalization. These processes decenter nations in the West as the only and dominant reference point for what it means to be modern and developed.

The Imaginaries and Cambodia in the Post-COVID World Order

While most of my fieldwork for this book took place between 2016 and 2019, I returned to Phnom Penh in the summers of 2023 and 2024 to see what changes the COVID-19 pandemic brought to the Cambodian development sector. In the summer of 2024, I spoke with Sophal, the director of an NGO that worked in HIV services but would soon be closing its doors. Sophal informs me that since 2001 he had run his organization with funding from the U.S., Australia, and European nations, but now the grants are fewer, and the competition for funding is too steep. He tells me, "The time of massive Western intervention in Cambodia . . . I think maybe we are seeing its ending." When I ask what he will do instead of running his NGO, Sophal reports he does not know yet, but he is considering starting a business with his brother-in-law.

Sophal's perception that Western funding to the development sector in Cambodia is eroding is echoed by numerous practitioners in Phnom Penh. Economic downturn due to COVID-19 made aid donors from most nations in the Global North cut back on funding, at least temporarily. Cambodian practitioners also express a sense that, after providing aid to Cambodia since the late 1990s, the focus of Western foreign aid donors is turning to more pressing humanitarian crises, like the conflicts in Ukraine and Gaza. They also perceive Western donors to be currently experiencing economic decline and a rise in isolationist political leaders, leading to less aid funding. Another NGO interviewee, Sotheary, states, "The West just is not as rich as it once was and there are other problems in the world, but here, that means many Cambodian NGOs will have to close."

Several practitioners report they believe at least one hundred NGOs have closed since 2020, even before the USAID shutdown. Many NGOs that were previously entirely dependent on Western funding have also turned to new funding models. They have set up paid consulting offerings to support their work or created social enterprises, like Rith in the previous chapter, to fund their NGOs. Practitioners report these practices can enable some NGOs to keep running, but often at a much smaller scale than before. Further adding to the changes Cambodians are experiencing, European donors and INGOs are pushing for "decolonization" of the development sector in the form of more local leadership and lessening donor directives.[1] While such directives are aimed at giving practitioners in recipient nations more power, in the current context of limited donor funding, several Cambodian practitioners interpret it as another way that the West is pulling back.

These events have strengthened many Cambodian practitioners' resolve that the future of development entails a turn towards Asia. While COVID-19 restricted funding from all donors in the Global North, funding from East Asian donors returned more rapidly than others. Several local NGO directors reported that, along with Western donors, they had begun looking for and acquiring funding from South Korea, Japan, Taiwan, and their Southeast Asian neighbors like Singapore and Thailand. China also continues to provide copious loans to Cambodia. A number of practitioners brought up concerns about the increasing political power of China in Cambodia, and the fact that Chinese aid will not support NGOs or social programming (Stallings and Kim 2017). One interviewee worried, "I don't know what will happen to civil society advocacy activities with the rise of Asian donors. That's why we still try to get funding from the European nations to support those kinds of activities."

Nevertheless, with the sense that the power of the West is waning, numerous practitioners are hoping other nations in the Asian region will replace some of the funding lost from long-standing Western donors. They have found new, innovative ways to go after emerging donors. For instance, one NGO created an antimalarial bug spray it could sell cheaply to villagers in order to get investments from Singaporean corporations, instead of submitting traditional grant applications. This NGO's director reports that even though NGOs might need to get more creative in gaining funding, he believes civil society in Cambodia will continue.

Cambodian practitioners are not alone in noticing the lessening of Western aid resources available to NGOs. As discussed in chapter 1, in the late 1980s there was a movement for international development and foreign aid to address, not just economic development, but social ills such as poverty, healthcare, and gender equality. To implement the increasing number of social aid projects, in the 1990s the number of NGOs grew exponentially, sometimes called the "NGO boom" era. Yet, in the past decade, funding sources for NGOs have been declining around the world (Kermani and Reandi 2023). There has been a shift, led by many Asian and emerging donors, away from the social aid model described above and back to an emphasis on economic growth (Chorev 2020; Mawdsley, Savage, and Kim 2014). This may mean these organizations are facing an era of "NGO bust" due to funding limitations (Worley 2024). Furthermore, as I write this conclusion in 2025, Trump has shut down USAID, which will further impact NGO funding.

Foreign Aid and International Development in the Changing Global Order

As of this book's writing, President Trump has further transformed aid by shutting down USAID, pulling out of the World Health Organization, and is threatening to defund the World Bank and the International Monetary Fund (IMF). While it is unknown if the USAID shutdown will continue or if his threats to the global banks will be realized, the changes are already impacting the foreign aid sector. The U.S. has historically been the world's largest foreign aid donor in terms of the amount of money given, providing 63 billion U.S. dollars in foreign aid assistance in 2024 alone.[2] It is also the top shareholder and contributor to the World Bank and the IMF and a key contributor to the United Nations. This financial leadership has come with privileges like the ability to organize global trade regimes in the U.S.'s favor, affordable access to essential resources, and influence in global institutions. Historically, the countries that fund development are powerful knowledge producers about the path nations should take towards development, influencing the design of the world order (McMichael and Weber 2022).

It is unknown whether Trump's USAID shutdown will hold or what new foreign aid policy the U.S. may put in place. Nevertheless, damage has already been done to the standing of the U.S. in the global development sector. USAID-funded health clinics have closed. USAID-funded programs to prevent the spread of infectious diseases like HIV and tuberculosis have ended around the world. Additionally, approximately 10,000 USAID employees are now without jobs. Many private firms and NGOs dependent on USAID funding will soon need to downsize or close their doors. There are now significant doubts around the world about the reliability of the U.S. as a foreign aid donor, its role as a global leader, and its authority over knowledge about what it means to be a developed nation (Anderson et al. 2025).

This means the findings of this book are particularly pertinent in the current global political moment of increasing polarization, isolationism, and regionalization (Radhakrishnan and Solari 2023). The U.S. exit from the international aid sector has left a power vacuum that China, and other nations in Asia, are actively trying to fill. The end of USAID funding means that, China is now one of the largest players when it comes to development funding. Chinese development funding and its major project, the One Belt One Road Initiative, does not play by the long-held norms of the global development community (Wyrod 2019). Its aim is to enhance economic connectivity between China and countries in Asia, Europe, and Africa by building extensive infrastructure like roads, railways, and ports. Its eventual goal in doing so is to boost trade, gain affordable access to resources, and promote China's economic influence across these regions.

Through the One Belt One Road Initiative, China invested $679 billion U.S. dollars on infrastructure projects in nearly 150 countries between 2013 and 2022. China is not the only Asian nation playing a key role in development. Another emerging economic leader, India is also increasing its development aid. Since 2000, India's Ministry of External Affairs has overseen financial assistance to over 65 countries worth over $48 billion U.S. dollars (Nainar 2024). Finally, Japan also remains an influential donor, the fourth largest in the OECD, and South Korea is the twenty-eighth largest donor in the OECD in relative terms (OECD 2020). Alongside aid coming from East and South Asia is the production of "deterritorialized" and transferable visions of Asian capitalism and developmental states, which provide alternatives to the weakening American model of neoliberalism and state retrenchment (Hoang, Cobb, and Lei 2017: 635). In this changing geopolitical context, through their use of the development imaginaries, Cambodian practitioners show us what these regional alternatives mean for actors in the Global South.

New Imaginations of Development in the Global South

However, Cambodia is not the only nation in the Global South where comparisons between Asia and the West are being used strategically to modify understandings about possible paths towards national advancement. To illustrate this, this conclusion will briefly examine the influence of an East Asian development model and the use of regional imaginaries in Vietnam and sub-Saharan Africa, particularly Ethiopia. Vietnam, Cambodia's neighbor, is the country that Japan provides the second largest amount of aid funding to (Myanmar is the first) and it is the nation to which South Korea provides the largest amount of aid funding. Japan and South Korea are also Vietnam's top providers of foreign direct investment (Stallings and Kim 2017).

Vietnam and China have a politically tense relationship over several historical issues, including Vietnam's invasion of Cambodia during the Chinese-supported Khmer Rouge regime and claims to the South China Sea/Eastern Sea. Nevertheless, China also contributes substantial loans to Vietnam, is in the top ten of its foreign direct investors, and is Vietnam's largest trade partner (Stallings and Kim 2017). However, it must also be noted, since 1991, USAID has contributed more than 155 million dollars in assistance to improve the quality of life for citizens of Vietnam (although this is no longer true as of January 2025) and the U.S. is also among the top ten foreign direct investors to the country (Stallings and Kim 2017; U.S. Department of State 2025).

In this context, it is not surprising that we see instances of Vietnamese people debating their nation's development trajectory through comparisons between the West and Asia. Discussing the consequences of increasing foreign investment and the soaring popularity of cultural products from Japan and South Korea, some Vietnamese citizens worry that Asia is "recolonizing" Vietnam by extracting economic resources and importing cultural products. However, comparing Asia and the West, others argue foreign direct investment is a good thing because East Asians "make things better than the West" (Do and Dinh 2018; Thomas 2004).

Many Vietnamese citizens also argue East Asian countries provide a better development model for Vietnam than traditional Western nation states (Do and Dinh 2018; Wike et al. 2014). Despite Vietnam and China's political tensions, in 2014, one-fifth of the Vietnamese population agreed that China was the best model for Vietnamese development over other developed nations (Welsh and Chang 2015). In discussing East Asia's economic power, Thomas (2004) notes that Vietnamese citizens find it empowering to "see faces like ours" on the global stage. These examples illustrate comparisons between the West and Asia are salient in the articulations of national advancement and self-understandings in Vietnam.

Not unlike the Cambodian practitioners in this book, there is also evidence regional development imaginaries are used strategically in Vietnam to negotiate ideas about economic development (Kim 2017; Hoang 2015). For example, Vietnamese developers and government officials understand that the "West" and "Asia" have fundamental differences when it comes to urban development. For this reason, in a strategy Kim (2017) calls "modal governance," Vietnamese developers and officials strategically offer two modes to attract foreign capital. The first mode, transparency governance, which largely serves the World Bank and Western investors, is transparent about land purchases and urban development. The other mode, opaque governance, conducts business through personal connections and is offered to Asian neighbors who prefer to operate outside of competition with Western investors. Additionally, Hoang (2014) reports the idea of a regional, "Pan-Asian modernity" appeals to many Vietnamese and East Asia businessmen and political elites, which sex workers in Ho Chi Minh City deliberately draw on in attracting clients (514). Consequently, it's likely that strategic negotiations of the "West" and "Asia" are present in many Southeast Asians' work and personal lives.

However, the development imaginaries do not resonate just in Southeast Asian nations. Rearticulations of development using comparisons between Asia and the West are starting to take place, not just in Asia, but all over the Global South. For example, China, Japan, and South Korea play a dominant role as aid donors and investors in sub-Saharan Africa. During the 2021 Forum on China-Africa Cooperation, China signed strategic partnership initiatives with 44 African governments and pledged 40 billion U.S. dollars in the next three years to the region. Additionally, over 10,000 Chinese firms are current operating in sub-Saharan Africa (House Committee on Foreign Affairs 2022). Finally, in 2023, it was estimated African countries had received around 22 billion U.S. dollars in loans and investments from China's One Belt One Road Initiative (De Kluiver 2024).

Aid from China to African nations has yielded mixed results (Fourie 2017; Wyrod 2019; Obeng-Odoom 2024). China brings its own growth model to Africa by setting up infrastructure and regulations to create industrial parks and special economic zones in Africa, as industrial parks played a key role in China's earlier economic success (Davies 2008). Such projects frequently meet the approval of local business owners and political elites, with whom the Chinese work closely, but can ignore or exacerbate the needs of local workers. Nevertheless, understanding Chinese aid and economic development in Africa requires a nuanced perspective. For instance, economic projects implemented by Chinese provincial governments may be less sensitive to worker needs than Chinese central-state-led projects (Wyrod 2019). China is also viewed differently in distinctive African nations, with Nigeria (82 percent approval rating) and Kenya (77 percent approval rating) having the highest positive ratings for China in the region (Nassanga and Makara 2014).

Japan's official development aid (ODA) contributions to sub-Saharan Africa have increased drastically since the early 2000s. In 2022, the Ministry of Foreign Affairs Japan announced that, through its public and private sector support, Japan will make a financial contribution of over 30 billion U.S. dollars to Africa in the next three years (Ministry of Foreign Affairs Japan 2022). While Japan's increased funding for Africa is likely in response to China's turn towards the region, African nations generally have a positive view of Japan, with 87 percent of residents surveyed in Cote d'Ivoire, South Africa, and Kenya reporting they believe their nation's relationship with Japan is friendly (Endo 2013; Ministry of Foreign Affairs Japan 2018).

South Korea is a newer donor to the region. Nevertheless, it hosted its first Korea-Africa Summit in 2024 and is currently promising to increase its aid to the African region to 9 billion U.S. dollars by 2030 (Eom 2024). In contrast, the U.S., which has long been a key donor in the areas of health and humanitarian aid to Africa (providing 12 billion dollars to sub-Saharan Africa in 2024 alone), recently cut the majority of its aid to the African region with the USAID shutdown (Adegoke 2025). However, the U.S. does remain an important foreign direct investor in the region, making up 13 percent of Africa's total FDI (Trends 2024).

In consequence, not unlike Cambodian practitioners, citizens of African nations see increasing interactions with East Asian donors and realignments in the global order as resources for redefining their nation's place in the world (Balogun 2020). For instance, Ethiopian elites are making a bid to dub Ethiopia the "China of Africa" (Fourie 2017: 133). They argue they will do so by following China's rise to global economic prominence through export-oriented industrialization and the establishment of industrial parks.

Political leaders in Ethiopia asked the China Association of Development Zones to oversee the writing of their own national industrial park strategy. Yet, Ethiopian elites do not follow the Chinese model wholesale, and instead strategically negotiate it. For example, they made policies that require zero liquid waste discharge and no dorms on the factory site in the Chinese-funded Hawassa industrial park, sometimes drawing on Western-based rights discourse to do so (Fourie 2017).

The cases of Vietnam and Ethiopia illustrate that, beyond Cambodia, regional comparisons between Asia and the West are also being used strategically, not wholesale, to define national paths towards development. When we consider these cases, we can see that Cambodian practitioners are contributing to a larger process in which actors across the Global South are using development imaginaries to rewrite global hierarchies and the social identities that exist within them. In doing so, it is likely actors in the Global South will modify global institutions and global development norms (Tsutsui 2018). They have certainly done so in the past.

For instance, in the 1960s, 120 Global South nations joined the non-aligned movement, which aimed to challenge the international order centered on the Soviet Union and the U.S. By the 1970s, due in large part to the mobilization of the nonaligned movement, the G77, or Group of 77, was formed at the United Nations. The G77, which still exists today, is a coalition of developing countries which aims to promote its members' collective economic interests and create an enhanced joint negotiating capacity. The G77 launched a political campaign for a New International Economic Order (NIEO). The NIEO demanded the restructuring of the global economy in a more equitable fashion. While the NIEO was never fully enacted, the leaders of the powerful G7 nations were forced to contend with the NIEO's demands (Bair 2015; McMichael and Weber 2021; Nicholls 2019).[3]

Additionally, when enough states in the Global South demand and implement a policy change, it can come to modify global regulations. Chorev (2012) illustrates this in the case of nations from the Global South forcing the rewriting of global intellectual property laws for HIV medications to address their affordability. These examples demonstrate that nations in the Global South have, and can, contest and redefine global power dynamics, playing an important role in global political and economic transformations.

The competing development imaginaries this book documents are already modifying donor institutions. For example, while donors from China,

Japan, and South Korea played a role in creating the Asian development imaginary, donors now employ rearticulations of these ideas coming out of the Global South (Otele 2023). JICA interviewees know Cambodians are drawn to the idea of regional advancement. They report purposely putting these ideas in project documents and using them in meetings. For instance, one JICA employee compares Phnom Penh after the Khmer Rouge to Hiroshima after the atomic bomb. He tells me he got the idea to do so after hearing Cambodian practitioners make this comparison. In this example, regional norms produced in Cambodia become part of the rhetoric of Japan's bilateral agency.

However, the shuttering of USAID may mean we are entering an era of even more limitations on NGO funding. China is not known to provide social aid or fund NGOs, and while Japan and South Korea do so, it is in a much more limited fashion than the U.S. (Stallings and Kim 2017). Future research must be open to the ways increasing funding from East Asia may restrict global civil society organizations, but also the new diverse forms civil society organizations may take to stay afloat or attract new funding, like the social enterprises and start-up businesses NGOs opened in Phnom Penh.

Localizing Multivocal Development Imaginaries

In the future, to examine the diverse consequences the development imaginaries may come to have for the global order, we must not lose sight of previous insights from studies of international development. It has been a prominent theme in research on aid work that a core set of global values orient the global development sector, like individualism, neoliberal economic policies, or sustainable development (Bernal and Grewal 2014; Boli and Thomas 1999; Kentikelenis and Seabrooke 2017; Wyrod 2019). Then foreign aid donors ostensibly work to implement these, within their own nation's priorities, and one of the ways they do so is through supporting INGOs to implement development projects. However, due to the "local" context of recipient nations, the outcomes of these development projects are "always unforeseeable—[projects] become real through the work of generating and translating interests, creating context by tying in supporters and so sustaining interpretations" (Mosse and Lewis 2006: 13). In essence, studies have proven again and again that global norms are multivocal.

This is because practitioners and beneficiaries in recipient nations interpret global norms in radically diverse ways. For instance, in her study of feminist technology NGOs in Costa Rica, Valle (2023) illustrates that donors push NGOs to implement the global norm, women's economic empowerment. Donors support women learning to use technology to become individual entrepreneurs that support their families, but without addressing systemic inequalities. In contrast, feminists in these organizations use the logic of care to build collective feminist solidarity, "defying technocapitalist paradigms of digital inclusion" (3). Development projects are cultural products that are coproduced with different outcomes in distinctive contexts (Mosse and Lewis 2006; Swidler and Watkins 2017).

Nevertheless, challenging the above global-local perspective dominant in previous studies of development, this book has illustrated "global" norms largely come out of the development agenda of the West. The development imaginaries demonstrate that actors in the Global South are now comparing regional models when interpreting and implementing foreign aid projects. Yet, having reached this conclusion, we can now see that in future studies we cannot lose sight of the fact that development projects will still be interpreted differently in particular locales. That is, we must attend to the continued importance of the coproduction of development and multivocality within this new regionalized foreign aid system.

INGO practitioners in Cambodia mobilize the imaginaries of Asia and the West strategically to make new meanings as they implement donor projects. In chapter 2, we see practitioners at Japan Services Asia utilize the idea that Asian nations should have strong developmental states, like Japan, to justify both masculine authority in medicine and a strong public health sector that provides services to all mothers free of charge. Yet, in chapter 3, they parse out the differences between Japan and China to argue that the "Asian" way should follow China in respecting traditional medicine and elder knowledge. Consequently, it is clear that, like the well-studied Western (previously known as global) imaginary, the Asian development imaginary, and the ways it will change global development institutions, cannot be understood without attending to the role actors in the Global South play in how it is enacted.

Multivocal Development Imaginaries and Women's Empowerment

All over the world, gender is deeply intertwined in a nation's aspirations for modernity as well as the preservation of its cultural traditions (Abu-Lughod 1998; Balogun 2020; Hoang 2015; Matlon 2022; Shu and Chen

2023). Take, for instance, the popularity of the hashtag #tradwife in America today. Women pursing the #tradwife lifestyle enact the "traditional" gender roles of American culture. They promote a lifestyle in which they are subservient stay-at-home wives for male breadwinners, taking particular care of their feminine appearance. Yet, #tradwives draw on the modern rhetoric of Western feminism by arguing it is their choice to leave the workforce and to use social media to convince other American women to fulfill traditional gender roles. Going further, many successful #tradwives also actually earn some income as social media influencers. The #tradwife blends schemas from dominant "traditional" gender norms in America alongside the modern narratives of choice and entrepreneurship in Western feminism (Radhakrishnan and Solari 2025).

This example illustrates two important processes. First, we can see in it that tradition is not opposed to modernity but is often an integral part of constructing visions of what the modern, in this case woman, is or should be (Chen 2010). Additionally, it documents that even women in America are finding ways to take issue with the version of women's empowerment that has been a key part of the imaginary of the West since the 1990s. This is the form of empowerment that emphasizes individual economic choices for women, instead of any sort of collective mobilization or systemic change. After the end of the Cold War, this version of women's empowerment was promoted alongside neoliberal economic policies. The idea that empowered, self-reliant women will save themselves and their families from poverty through entrepreneurship has legitimized Western modernity. It does so by providing a "choice" to bridge the gap between women's (and the nation's) aspirations and the lived realities of an unequal global economy (Radhakrishnan and Solari 2023; Rankin 2001; Valle 2023).

But it is becoming increasingly clear that this version of women's empowerment has not resulted in a world of gender egalitarianism (Radhakrishnan and Solari 2023). Women around the world are still more likely to be in poverty and take up the majority of household and childcare labor (UN Women 2023). Even for American women, it is not easy to "do it all." America women are burned out from pursuing career success while often continuing to take on the majority of childcare and household labor, and, in the case of the #tradwife, are willing to valorize patriarchal structures if it means they get to do less (Radhakrishnan and Solari 2025).

As we see the #tradwives do, Cambodian practitioners use the development imaginaries to blend different schemas about what is modern and traditional throughout this book, particularly when discussing men's and women's roles in society. In this process, the Asian development imaginary is employed with mixed results for women's empowerment and gender equality. On the one hand, Japan Services Asia's program managers draw on traditional beliefs that women's place is in the home to justify that men are breadwinners and women's income is secondary. This is enabled by the fact that East Asian foreign aid donors are less likely to integrate gender equality trainings or measures into their aid projects (Zhang and Huang 2023). The lack of discussion about gender inequality gives practitioners more opportunities to use the Asian imaginary to reinforce gender norms that relegate women to the home and childcare.

Yet, also in chapter 4, we saw practitioners at U.S. Family Aid employ the Asian imaginary to challenge the Western notion that all workers should be treated equally, because it ignores the unique challenges faced by mothers with young children. Cambodian practitioners argue that in Asian families the mothers of young children are respected. They contend there is a need for workplace policies to be put in place that create accommodations for mothers. Consequently, this book illustrates that the imaginary of Asia, just like the imaginary of the West, can be used in ways that both discourage and benefit gender equality. Such a finding is in line with what feminists of the Global South have long argued. We cannot assume the West's ideas about gender equality are immediately more liberatory than gendered beliefs available in nations in the Middle East, Africa, or Asia.

As development imaginaries are multivocal, the ways that they may be used to realign domestic and global gender inequalities is not a foregone conclusion. We can see this if we return to the conversation at the USAID workshop from the introduction to this book. The speaker introduces the question—"How can we strive for women's empowerment and preserve our culture at the same time?" One NGO practitioner responds, "If we take up all these Western ideas about gender like USAID wants us to—how will we still be Cambodian? Asia must make its own way." Another NGO director responds passionately, "What do you mean by culture and tradition? . . . if what you mean by culture is that we celebrate Khmer New Year, bring food to the monks, wear special clothes, then that's nice. But culture is often used to oppress women. We are not destroying culture by women having more freedom. We need to have a dialogue about what is culture and how can women's equality be part of it in Asia."

In this conversation it is now clear gender is deeply embedded in contestations of Western dominance, ideas about what will make for a "modern" Asia, and the construction of a new world order. Yet it is also evident that practitioners in Cambodia are still deciding what the role of gender will be in "modern Asia." We are living in a moment of global transition, and actors in Cambodia, and throughout the Global South, are actively engaged in debating the future of gender equality in development.

Such debates are pressing in the current historical moment of increasing gender backlash. The rise in populist and isolationist rhetoric has been accompanied by an increase in gender equality backlash and masculine authority (Radhakrishnan and Solari 2025). In this context, development practitioners and international activists who are interested in global gender equality or transnational feminist organizing might use the development imaginaries "as a springboard into imagining and creating alternative futures" (Mohan and Stokke 2000: 262). As we saw U.S. Family Aid practitioners do in chapter 4, it is certainly possible to draw on schemas in the Asian imaginary, like collectivism, respect, the importance of family and community, or even socioeconomic prosperity for all, to push back on or hybridize the dominant individualistic model of women's economic empowerment. Consequently, the Asian imaginary could be of assistance in valorizing collectivist projects, like reimagining women's empowerment, and taking a step towards building a more equitable world.[4]

Methodological Appendix
Aid Chain Ethnography and Feminist Reflections

Ethnography and the Self

To conduct an ethnography across multiple sites requires the construction of multiple social selves. During fieldwork, I spent months living in the urban centers of Washington, D.C., Tokyo, and Phnom Penh, but also in rural towns in the Cambodian provinces of Kampong Speu and Steung Treng. In each site, I highlighted different aspects of my own social self to gain rapport and social acceptance. In Tokyo, my academic credentials were often front and center in interactions with development workers. In Washington, D.C., what mattered most were my experiences as an NGO worker and development consultant.

In Phnom Penh, I befriended female NGO staff through shared experiences of "modern girl" time such as getting our nails done, shopping, or going out for coffee, drinks, or food. In Steung Treng and Kampong Speu, my academic credentials meant little. Many villagers were interested in stories about and photos of my family, my home, and sharing stories of theirs, as well as laughing at my inability to drive a manual transmission motor scooter successfully or the fact that the water buffalo were terrified of me. I left the field with a deep, sometimes disorienting sense of one of the basic teachings from Introduction to Sociology: identity, how we define and understand ourselves, is so deeply based on the social groups we are in.

This social shifting enabled me to make friends in each field site. I am deeply indebted to all of them for sharing their stories of how they negotiate their work and their identities. And, of course, within these interactions, it was crucial to take stock of how my own shifting position impacted the data I could collect and how I would interpret it. As feminist and postcolonial scholarship points out, all knowledge comes from a perspective, and each of us must reflect carefully on how our own position and perspective shapes the knowledge we create (Mies 1979; Mohanty 1988; Naples 2017). Following feminist methodologies, I paid careful attention to positionality and the power dynamics that came alongside it throughout my fieldwork.

In interactions with Cambodian practitioners, as a white American, I immediately am often assumed to have expert development knowledge, access to resources, and perhaps some sort of influence over donors. When they heard about my project, which provided me with the privilege of traveling to Tokyo, Washington, D.C., and Cambodia, the perception that I had access to resources and connections with donors increased. This outsider status inevitably shaped Cambodians' interaction patterns with me, and it took time to get past deferential interactions. However, I conducted the fieldwork for this text in Cambodia over the summers of 2016, 2017, 2023, 2024, and the 2018–19 school year. Time spent in the field and conversational Khmer language skills assisted me in getting to know participants and building their trust over time. Additionally, some participants were more likely to complain and explain donor practices to me in the interest of assisting me in "getting it right" for my research project.

In Washington, D.C., my positionality shifted to somewhat "insider" status, as someone who had worked in NGOs and an American. This enabled me to speak the language needed to gain rapport quickly, but it also required me to take a beginner's mindset in Washington, D.C., so as not to rely on my own taken-for-granted assumptions. Finally, in Tokyo, I found development practitioners quite eager to talk to an academic about their work, as many NGOs are marginalized, small charities in Japan. In the development sector, most practitioners spoke English, but I did need a translator to observe development events. Also, visits from headquarters staff to Cambodia allowed me to know several Japanese headquarters staff members over time and form friendships.

However, in my Tokyo case, I had to pay careful attention to my own assumptions about development, gender, and the state/market/civil society matrix. It was only through coffees and in-depth conversations with key informants that I got a sense of the different definitions global development vocabulary can have in Japan. My more limited experience with the language and culture in Japan also restricted my gaining a deeper understanding of the ways development work impacted their identities. I was careful to note this, and it is why the book focuses largely on Cambodian practitioners' identity work, as this is the context where I spent the most time getting to know practitioners.

In each ethnographic site, my positionality shifted, requiring analysis of how this enabled and constrained the type of data I was able to collect. Inevitably, my position and work in each organization also modified the worksites themselves to a small extent. I often traded personal skills and labor to gain research access to the organizations. At my local NGO field site in Kampong Speu, which I call Cambodian Development Society, I assisted in completely rewriting their English mission statement and annual reports, altering how the NGO was perceived by English readers to some degree. At U.S. Family Aid in Phnom Penh, I assisted with research for their gender analysis, modifying the types of gender equality activities integrated into their future programs. In each case, I gave back to the organization in whatever way was requested, taking part in the construction of development in workplace interactions, the very thing I was studying.

Aid Chains and the Analysis of Power

Feminist scholars and methodologists promote a careful analysis of power in one's research site, both in terms of how it impacts the research and how it can be studied. Some argue for the importance of bringing those "at the margins to the center" to better understand the social world (hooks 1984). Yet, this can leave a power differential between those conducting research and those "being researched." Other feminist scholars argue for a careful analysis of those with power and resources, revealing the processes through which power works and is upheld. This can alleviate some of the above power inequalities between researcher and researched. However, it can also reify the center and its power instead of decentering it.

Following Shih (2023), this book works to combine these two perspectives through "studying across." Through analysis of aid chains, I observe those with material resources and ideational influence in the chain, that is, donors and headquarter organizations. And I also observe the interactions between those in powerful positions and practitioners as well as beneficiaries in the Global South. In the study of how imaginaries are strategically employed, I center the voices of practitioners in the Global South who are challenging and modifying, instead of reifying, the work of donors and INGOs in powerful nations. In doing so, the book analyzes both powerful foreign aid institutions and the actors in the Global South that are remaking them.

Notes

Introduction

1. Cambodian people's culture is called Khmer.

2. After the prime minister disbanded the opposition party, most Western donors discontinued aid to the Cambodian elections and spoke out against the 2018 election in Cambodia for not being free and fair. After immense pressure from other donors, Japan also pulled out of election funding just days before it took place, but remained publicly silent on why it did so.

3. I acknowledge the use of the term "Global South" has deep limitations as it tries to capture in one catchall term an array of nations that differ markedly. However, the term has been appealing to and is used by many lower- and middle-income countries as a political term used to address enduring global hierarchies and inequalities. It is in this spirit that I use "Global South" in this book—not as a rigid grouping or homogenization of the nations within it—but as an organizing concept for reimagining the world order (Hogan and Patrick 2024).

4. Whether NGOs should be implicitly considered civil society organizations is up for debate (Brass 2016). USAID uses the rhetoric of civil society support when it funds NGOs, so the term is used here.

5. While China would be an interesting case, this book examines social development projects implemented by INGOs and, at the time of this research, China did not fund NGOs in Cambodia.

6. For reference, the U.S. is ranked 43 and Japan is ranked 118.

7. The exact location of each field site has also been modified for anonymity.

Chapter 1

1. Just because feminist groups allied with them, we cannot assume that nationalist and anticolonialist movements always had feminist aims. Notions of "traditional" womanhood were often used by these movements to construct national ideals (Puri 2003).

2. It must be noted that the term "gender" itself has a racialized and colonial history in its construction in the U.S. academic context; and globalization of the term is inextricably bound up with U.S. global hegemony (Patil 2022).

Chapter 2

1. See https://www.un.org/en/sections/resources-different-audiences/civil-society/index.html.

2. Not all communes have a health center as it depends on their geographic size and population.

3. Only 23 percent of doctors in Japan itself are women and even fewer women are public health officials (Nippon 2024). In Cambodia, while the share of female public health workers is increasing, leadership positions are still highly male-dominated (Vong et al. 2019).

4. For comparison, the German bilateral agency, GIZ, might be considered a bilateral development agency that closely resembles JICA, since it also implements the majority of its programming in close cooperation with the Cambodian state. GIZ also funds and implements maternal and child health projects in Cambodia. To do so, GIZ also employed the train-the-trainers model, working directly with provincial hospital doctors to train midwives on emergency obstetric care. Additionally, though, GIZ engages local NGOs to provide health trainings directly to local communities in order to, as one GIZ official reports, "build Cambodian civil society." In contrast, JSA provides health trainings solely to government health staff.

5. Khmer language does not use the roman alphabet. All transliterations are my own.

6. "Health behavior change communication" is a health communication technique used in international development; see https://healthcommcapacity.org/about/why-social-and-behavior-change-communication/.

7. "Human-centered design" is an iterative design process that works to understand the people who use a product or service to solve their problems; see https://www.designkit.org/human-centered-design.

8. For the purposes of comparison with JSA's JICA-funded health project, this research focuses on USFA's largest project, its USAID-funded health project to promote health behavior change. Yet even when narrowing my discussion of USFA to a single project, the organization's larger size and complexity compared to JSA

makes the comparison inexact. The budget for USFA's health behavior change project is substantially larger than JSA's project ($10 million vs. $1 million U.S. dollars) and the single project has multiple goals that involve diverse partnerships.

9. These claims are made even though programming that encourages democracy is rarely pursued by Japanese development organizations, and South Korea also provides aid in Africa.

Chapter 3

1. U.S. Family Aid (USFA) subgrants to the local NGO, Cambodian Development Society (CDS), to implement USFA's maternal health and family planning activities in Kampong Speu. In doing so, USFA re-creates a relationship with CDS very similar to the one it has with USAID. It calls for proposals from local NGOs and, after CDS wins the project, USFA and CDS enter a contract, which details the specific activities CDS will implement and the measurable outcomes that will be produced.

2. This contrasts with many European-funded women's health organizations I interviewed, which reported creating women's health advocacy groups.

3. Factory workers are a group considered in particular need of reproductive health information.

4. Unlike JSA, foreign staff at USFA recognize it is not possible to provide only biomedical information to mothers and encourage CDS staff to discuss traditional practices. They discourage a few harmful ones, like the practice of roasting, where newborns and mothers sit over hot coals. But other practices, such as prayers or offerings to ancestors or spirits, are encouraged alongside biomedical care practices (Bazzano et al. 2020).

5. Reasmey reports CDS staff always tell women about the abortion laws in Cambodia, even though their donor rules and regulations around that sometimes change due to USAID's implementation and lifting of the Mexico City Policy discussed in chapter 1.

Chapter 4

1. When Junko, Hanako, or headquarters staff are present, workplace conversations are conducted in English, but otherwise staff members speak Khmer among themselves. On occasion, clarifications are made in Khmer, which Junko also speaks.

Chapter 5

1. Of course, this budget does not exist since USAID's shutdown, which will be discussed in depth in the conclusion.

Chapter 6

1. Gold came to Cambodia from China or other Southeast Asian empires; it is not native to Cambodia.

2. While USFA staff work on two different teams, monitoring and evaluation or project management, there is not a significant difference in the motivations or class status of workers at USFA.

3. As monks are not allowed to deal with money, he could not remain a monk and direct an NGO.

Conclusion

1. See, e.g., Oxfam's report on decolonization: https://policy-practice.oxfam.org/resources/decolonize-what-does-it-mean-621456/.

2. It must be noted that although the U.S. gives the most foreign aid assistance in sheer amount of money, we only give 0.2 percent of our gross national product (GNP). Many nations in the Global North give more. For instance, Sweden gives 1 percent of its GNP (Ingram 2019).

3. The Group of Seven (G7) is made up of Canada, France, Germany, Italy, Japan, the United Kingdom, and the United States. The European Union is also a nonenumerated member.

4. The Asian imaginary, as practitioners in this text have used it, is deeply limited in its liberatory capacity by the lack of engagement with sexuality and gender-nonconforming people.

References

Abu-Lughod, Lila. 1998. *Remaking Women: Feminism and Modernity in the Middle East*. Princeton University Press.

Acker, Joan. 1990. "Hierarchies, Jobs, Bodies: A Theory of Gendered Organizations." *Gender and Society* 4 (2): 139–58.

Adegoke, Yinka. 2025. "Seven African Countries to Be Hit Hardest by Trump USAID Cuts." *Semafor*. https://www.semafor.com/article/02/12/2025/countries -worst-hit-by-usaid-cuts.

Akpan, Wilson. 2011. "Local Knowledge, Global Knowledge, Development Knowledge: Finding a Balance in the Knowledge Power Play." *South African Review of Sociology* 42 (3): 116–27.

Alexander, Jacqui. 2006. *Pedagogies of Crossing: Meditations on Feminism, Sexual Politics, Memory, and the Sacred*. Duke University Press.

Almeling, Rene. 2007. "Selling Genes, Selling Gender: Egg Agencies, Sperm Banks, and the Medical Market in Genetic Material." *American Sociological Review* 72 (3): 319–40.

Alvarez, Sonia E. 2009. "Beyond NGO-ization? Reflections from Latin America." *Development* 52 (2): 175–84.

Anderson, Elizabeth, and Kelly Grace. 2018. "From Schoolgirls to 'Virtuous' Khmer Women: Interrogating Chbab Srey and Gender in Cambodian Education Policy." *Studies in Social Justice* 12 (2): 215–34.

Anderson, Scott, Vanda Felbab-Brown, Michael Hansen, George Ingram, Thomas

Pepinsky, Anthony Pipa, Molly Reynolds, Sweta Shah, and Landry Singe. 2025. "The Implications of the USAID Shutdown." *Brookings Institution.* https://www.brookings.edu/articles/what-comes-after-a-usaid-shutdown/.

Arase, David, ed. 2005. *Japan's Foreign Aid: Old Continuities and New Directions.* Routledge.

Arellano, Janice. 2015. "Don't Leave U.S. Behind: Problems with the Existing Family and Medical Leave Act, and Alternatives to Help Enhance the Employee Work-Family Relationship in the 21st Century." *Journal of Workplace Rights* 5 (2): 1–13.

Arrighi, Giovanni. 2009. *Adam Smith in Beijing.* Verso.

Asia Development Bank. 2014. "Country Partnership Strategy 2014–2018: Gender Analysis." https://www.adb.org/sites/default/files/linked-documents/cps-cam-2014-2018-ga.pdf.

Atlani-Duault, Laetitia. 2007. *Humanitarian Aid in Post-Soviet Countries: An Anthropological Perspective.* Routledge.

Babb, Sarah, and Alexander Kentikelenis. 2021. "Markets Everywhere: The Washington Consensus and the Sociology of Global Institutional Change." *Annual Review of Sociology* 47: 521–41.

Bair, Jennifer. 2015. "Corporations at the United Nations: Echoes of the New International Economic Order?" *Humanity: An International Journal of Human Rights, Humanitarianism, and Development* 6 (1): 159–71.

Balogun, Oluwakemi. 2020. *Beauty Diplomacy: Embodying an Emerging Nation.* Stanford University Press.

Banchani, Emmanuel, and Liam Swiss. 2019. "The Impact of Foreign Aid on Maternal Mortality." United Nation's University WIDER Working Paper.

Bandelj, Nina. 2020. "Relational Work in the Economy." *Annual Review of Sociology* 46: 251–72.

Banks, Nicola, David Hulme, and Michael Edwards. 2015. "NGOs, States, and Donors Revisited: Still Too Close for Comfort?" *World Development* 66:707–18.

Barot, Sneha. 2017. "The Benefits of Investing in International Family Planning—and the Price of Slashing Funding." *Guttmacher Policy Review* 20: 82–85.

Barr, Michael D. 2002. *Cultural Politics and Asian Values.* Routledge.

Bazzano, Alessandra N., Jeni Stolow, Ryan Duggal, Richard Oberhelman, and Chivorn Var. 2020. "Warming the Postpartum Body as a Form of Postnatal Care: An Ethnographic Study of Medical Injections and Traditional Health Practices in Cambodia." *PLoS One,* 15 (2): 1–16.

Bernal, Victoria, and Inderpal Grewal, eds. 2014. *Theorizing NGOs: States, Feminisms, and Neoliberalism.* Duke University Press.

Benzecry, Claudio. 2022. *The Perfect Fit: Creative Work in the Global Shoe Industry.* University of Chicago Press.

Black, Lindsay. 2017. "Japan's Aspirations for Regional Leadership—Is the Goose Finally Cooked?" *Japanese Studies* 37 (2): 151–70.

Blair, Robert, Robert Marty, and Phillip Roessler. 2022. "Foreign Aid and Soft Power: Great Power Competition in Africa in the Early Twenty-first Century." *British Journal of Political Science* 52:1355–76.

Boli, John, and George Thomas, eds. 1999. *Constructing World Culture: International Nongovernmental Organizations Since 1875*. Stanford University Press.

Boling, Patricia. 2015. *The Politics of Work-Family Policies: Comparing Japan, France, Germany and the United States*. Cambridge University Press.

Boserup, Ester. 1970. *Women's Role in Economic Development*. Earthscan.

Bracke, Maud Anne. 2023. "Contesting 'Global Sisterhood': The Global Women's Health Movement, the United Nations and the Different Meanings of Reproductive Rights." *Gender and History* 35 (3): 769–1165.

Brass, Jennifer N. 2016. *Allies or Adversaries: NGOs and the State in Kenya*. Cambridge University Press.

Brass, Jennifer N. 2021. "Do Service Provision NGOs Perform Civil Society Functions? Evidence of NGOs' Relationship with Democratic Participation." *Nonprofit and Voluntary Sector Quarterly* 51 (1): 148–69.

Brickell, Katherine. 2011. " 'We Don't Forget the Old Rice Pot When We Get the New One': Discourses on Ideals and Practices of Women in Contemporary Cambodia." *Signs* 36 (2): 437–62.

Bromley, Patricia, Evan Schofer, and Wesley Longhofer. 2019. "Contentions over World Culture: The Rise of Legal Restrictions on Foreign Funding to NGOs, 1994–2015." *Social Forces* 99 (1): 281–304.

Caballero, Paula. 2019. "The SDGs: Changing How Development Is Understood." *Global Policy* 10 (1): 138–40.

Cambodia Demographic and Health Survey. 2014. Ministry of Planning, National Institute of Statistics and Ministry of Health Directorate General for Health and Measure DHS. https://dhsprogram.com/pubs/pdf/FR377/FR377.pdf.

Cambodian Cooperation Committee. 2020. "CSO Database." https://www.ccc-cambodia.org/en/ngodb/ngo-information.

Carpenter, Laura, and Monica Casper. 2009. "A Tale of Two Technologies: HPV Vaccination, Male Circumcision, and Sexual Health." *Gender and Society* 23 (6): 790–816.

Chandler, David. 2007. *A History of Cambodia*. 4th ed. Routledge.

Channyda, Chenda. 2017. "Commune Elections 2017: CPP Wins 70%." *Phnom Penh Post*. http://www.phnompenhpost.com/national-post-depth-politics/cpp-wins-70-communes.

Chen, Kuan-Hsing. 2010. *Asia as Method: Toward Deimperialization*. Duke University Press.

Chorev, Nitsan. 2012. *The World Health Organization Between North and South.* Cornell University Press.

Chorev, Nitsan. 2019. *Give and Take: Developmental Foreign Aid and the Pharmaceutical Industry in East Africa.* Princeton University Press.

Chu, Yin-Wah, ed. 2016. *The Asian Developmental State.* Palgrave Macmillan.

Ciccantell, Paul, and Stephen Bunker. 2004. "The Economic Ascent of China and the Potential for Restructuring the Capitalist World-Economy." *Journal of World-System Research* 3: 565–89.

Cold-Ravnkilde, Signe Marie, Lars Engberg-Pedersen, and Adam Moe Fejerskov. 2018. "Global Norms and Heterogenous Development Organizations." *Progress in Development Studies* 18 (2): 77–94.

Connell, R. W. 1990. "The State, Gender, and Sexual Politics: Theory and Appraisal." *Theory and Society* 19 (5): 507–44.

Connell, R. W. 2012. "Gender, Health and Theory: Conceptualizing the Issue, in Local and World Perspective." *Social Science and Medicine* 74 (11): 1675–83.

Council for the Development of Cambodia. 2024. "Employment and Labor." Royal Government of Cambodia. https://cdc.gov.kh/laws-and-regulations/employment-and-labor/.

Cummins, Emily R., and Linda M. Blum. 2015. " 'Suits to Self-Sufficiency': Dress for Success and Neoliberal Maternalism." *Gender and Society* 29 (5): 623–46.

Cupac, Jelena, and Irem Tuncer-Ebeturk. 2022. "Competitive Mimicry: The Socialization of Antifeminist NGOs into the United Nations." SSRN. *Global Constitutionalism*, 1–22.

Das, Devaleena. 2023. "What Transnational Feminism Has Not Disrupted Yet." *Meridians* 22 (2): 240–66.

Davies, Martyn. 2008. "China's Developmental Model Comes to Africa." *Review of African Political Economy* 35 (115): 134–37.

Davis, Kathy. 2007. *The Making of 'Our Bodies, Ourselves': How Feminism Travels Across Borders.* Duke University Press.

Decoteau, Claire Laurier. 2013. *Ancestors and Antiretrovirals: The Biopolitics of HIV/ AIDS in Post-Apartheid South Africa.* University of Chicago Press.

De Kluiver, Jana. 2024. "Africa Has Much to Gain from a More Contained BRI." Institute for Security Studies. https://issafrica.org/iss-today/africa-has-much-to-gain-from-a-more-contained-bri.

Delbanco, Suzzane, Maclaine Lehan, Thi Montalvo, and Jeffery Levin-Scherz. 2019. "The U.S. Maternal Mortality Rate Demands Action from Employers." *Harvard Business Review.* https://hbr.org/2019/06/the-rising-u-s-maternal-mortality-rate-demands-action-from-employers.

Derks, Annuska. 2008. *Khmer Women on the Move: Exploring Work and Life in Urban Cambodia.* University of Hawaii Press.

Desai, Manisha. 2015. "Critical Cartography, Theories, and Praxis of Transnational

Feminisms." In *The Oxford Handbook of Transnational Feminist Movements*, ed. Rawwida Baksh and Wendy Harcourt, chap. 4. Oxford University Press.

DeVault, Marjorie. 1996. "Talking Back to Sociology: Distinctive Contributions of Feminist Methodology." *Annual Review of Sociology* 22: 29–50.

Dietrich, Simone. 2021. *States, Markets, and Foreign Aid*. Cambridge University Press.

Dingle, Antonia, Timothy Powell-Jackson, and Catherine Goodman. 2013. "A Decade of Improvements in Equity of Access to Reproductive and Maternal Health Services in Cambodia, 2000–2010." *International Journal for Equity in Health* 12: 51.

Dionne, Kim Yi. 2018. *Doomed Interventions: The Failure of Global Responses to AIDS in Africa*. Cambridge University Press.

Do, Thuy T., and Julia Luong Dinh. 2018. "Vietnam-Japan Relations: Moving Beyond Economic Cooperation?" In *Vietnam's Foreign Policy Under Doi Moi*, ed. H. H. Le and A. Tsvetov, 96–116. Lectures, Workshops, and Proceedings of International Conferences. ISEAS–Yusof Ishak Institute.

Dromi, Shai M. 2016. "For Good and Country: Nationalism and the Diffusion of Humanitarianism in the Late Nineteenth Century." *Sociological Review* 64 (2): 79–97.

Ear, Sophal. 2013. *Aid Dependence in Cambodia: How Foreign Assistance Undermines Democracy*. Columbia University Press.

Egan, John, and Santhosh Persaud. 2021. "12 Ways Korea Is Changing the World: From Emerging Donor to Global Development Partner." OECD Report. https://www.oecd.org/country/korea/thematic-focus/from-emerging-donor-to-global-development-partner-66044045/.

Ellwood, Marilyn Rymer, and Genevieve Kenney. 1995. "Medicaid and Pregnant Women: Who Is Being Enrolled and When." *Healthcare Financing Review* 17 (2): 7–28.

Endo, Mitsugui. 2013. "From 'Reactive' to 'Principled': Japan's Foreign Policy Stance Towards Africa." Japan's Diplomacy Series, Japan Digital Library. https://www2.jiia.or.jp/en/pdf/digital_library/japan_s_diplomacy/160330_Mitsugi_Endo.pdf.

Eom, Tae Yeon. 2024. "Why Africa Matters to South Korea's Indo-Pacific Strategy." *Asia Pacific Foundation of Canada*. https://www.asiapacific.ca/publication/why-africa-matters-south-koreas-indo-pacific-strategy#:~:text=South%20Korea's%20official%20development%20assistance,Korean%20companies%20operating%20in%20Africa.

Er, Lam Peng. 2013. *Japan's Relations with Southeast Asia: The Fukuda Doctrine and Beyond*. Routledge.

Escobar, Arturo. 1995. *Encountering Development: The Making and Unmaking of the Third World*. Princeton University Press.

Estevez-Abe, Margarita. 2014. "An International Comparison of Institutional Requisites for Gender Equality." *Japanese Economy* 39 (3): 77–98.

Fahlberg, Anjuli. 2023. *Activism Under Fire: The Politics of Non-Violence in Rio De Janeiro's Gang Territories.* Oxford University Press.

Fechter, Anne-Meike. 2019. "Brokering Transnational Flows of Care: The Case of Citizen Aid." *Ethnos* 85: 293–309.

Fengxian, Wang. 2012. "The 'Good Wife and Wise Mother' as a Social Discourse of Gender." Chinese Studies in History 45 (4): 58–70.

Ferguson, Jason L. 2021. " 'There Is an Eye on Us': International Imitation, Popular Representation, and the Regulation of Homosexuality in Senegal." *American Sociological Review* 86 (4): 700–727.

Fernandes, Sujatha. 2017. "Stories and Statecraft: Afghan Women's Narratives and the Construction of Western Freedoms." *Signs* 42 (3): 643–67.

Ferree, Myra M., and Aili M. Tripp, eds. 2006. *Global Feminism.* New York University Press.

FHI360. 2010. The Essential NGO Guide to Managing Your USAID Award. https://www.fhi360.org/wp-content/uploads/drupal/documents/Essential Guide.pdf.

Fourcade-Gourinchas, Marion, and Sarah L. Babb. 2002. "The Rebirth of the Liberal Creed: Paths to Neoliberalism in Four Countries." *American Journal of Sociology* 108 (3): 533–79.

Fourie, Elsje. 2017. "The Intersection of East Asian and African Modernities: Towards a New Research Agenda." *Social Imaginaries* 3 (1): 119–46.

Frank, David, Wesley Longhofer, and Evan Schofer. 2007. "World Society, NGOs and Environmental Policy Reform in Asia." *International Journal of Comparative Sociology* 48 (4): 275–95.

Frewer, Tim. 2013. "Doing NGO Work: The Politics of Being 'Civil Society' and Promoting 'Good Governance' in Cambodia." *Australian Geographer* 44 (1): 97–114.

Frieson, Kate. 2001. "In the Shadows: Women, Power, and Politics in Cambodia." Centre for Asia-Pacific Initiatives, Occasional Paper No. 26.

Frieson, Kate, Men Chean, Socheat Chi, Hou Nirmita, and Chev Mony. 2011. "A Gender Analysis of the Cambodian Health Sector." AusAid, Final Research Report. https://dfat.gov.au/about-us/publications/Documents/health-sector -gender-analysis.pdf.

Fujimura-Fanselow, Kumiko. 2014. "The Japanese Ideology of 'Good Wives and Wise Mothers': Trends in Contemporary Research." *Gender and History* 3 (3): 345–49.

Ganti, Tejaswini. 2014. "Neoliberalism." *Annual Review of Anthropology* 43: 89–104.

Garita, Alexandra. 2015. "Moving Toward Sexual and Reproductive Justice: A

Transnational and Multigenerational Feminist Remix." In *The Oxford Handbook of Transnational Feminist Movements*, ed. Rawwida Baksh and Wendy Harcourt, chap. 10. Oxford University Press.

Gavalyugova, Dimitria, and Wendy Cunningham. 2020. "Gender Analysis of the Cambodian Labor Market." World Bank Publications, Reports 34201, World Bank Group.

Gibson, Megan. 2015. "The Long, Strange History of Birth Control." *Time Magazine*. https://time.com/3692001/birth-control-history-djerassi/.

Giordano, Chiara. 2019. "The Role of Gender Regimes in Defining the Dimension, the Functioning and the Workforce Composition of Paid Domestic Work." *Feminist Review* 122 (1): 95–117.

Goetz, Anna Marie. 2020. "The New Competition in International Norm Setting: Transnational Feminists and the Illiberal Backlash." *American Academy of Arts and Sciences Creative Commons*. https://www.amacad.org/sites/default/files/publication/downloads/Daedalus_Wi20_11_Goetz_0.pdf.

Greenhill, Romilly, Annalisa Prizzon, and Andrew Rogerson. 2016. "The Age of Choice: Developing Countries in the New Aid Landscape." In *The Fragmentation of Aid*, ed. S. Klingebiel, T. Mahn, and M. Negre, 137–51. Palgrave Macmillan.

Grewal, Inderpal. 1996. *Home and Harem: Nation, Gender, Empire, and the Cultures of Travel*. Duke University Press.

Grewal, Inderpal, and Caren Kaplan. 2002. *Scattered Hegemonies: Postmodernity and Transnational Feminist Practices*. University of Minnesota Press.

Gunja, Munira, Evan Gumas, Relebohile Masitha, and Laurie Zephyrin. 2024. "Insights into the U.S. Maternal Mortality Crisis." Commonwealth Fund. Issue Briefs. https://www.commonwealthfund.org/publications/issue-briefs/2024/jun/insights-us-maternal-mortality-crisis-international-comparison.

Gunja, Murina, Evan Gumas, and Reginald Williams. 2023. "U.S. Health Care from a Global Perspective, 2022: Accelerating Spending, Worsening Outcomes." Commonwealth Fund. https://www.commonwealthfund.org/publications/issue-briefs/2023/jan/us-health-care-global-perspective-2022.

Hall, Rodney. 2003. "The Discursive Demolition of the Asian Development Model." *International Studies Quarterly* 47 (1): 71–99.

Halliday, Terence, and Bruce Carruthers. 2009. *Bankrupt: Global Lawmaking and Systemic Financial Crisis*. Stanford University Press.

Hammack, David C. 2002. "Nonprofit Organizations in American History." *American Behavioral Scientist* 45 (11): 1638–74.

Hart, Gillian. 2002. *Disabling Globalization: Places of Power in Post-Apartheid South Africa*. University of California Press.

Hays, Sharon. 1998. *The Cultural Contradictions of Motherhood*. Yale University Press.

Heidenreich, Martin. 2012. "State of the Art: The Social Embeddedness of Multinational Companies: A Literature Review." *Socioeconomic Review* 10 (3): 549–79.

Helfen, Markus, Elke Schüßler, and Dimitris Stevis. 2016. "Translating European Labor Relations Practices to the United States Through Global Framework Agreements? German and Swedish Multinationals Compared." *ILR Review* 69 (3): 631–55.

Heng, Geraldine. 2018. *The Invention of Race in the European Middle Ages*. Cambridge University Press.

Higuchi, Toshihiro. 2013. "How US Aid in the 1950s Prepared Japan as a Future Donor." In *The Rise of Asian Donors: Japan's Impact on the Evolution of Emerging Donors*, ed. J. Sato and Y. Shimomura. Routledge.

Hirata, Keiko. 2002. *Civil Society in Japan: The Growing Role of NGOs in Tokyo's Aid and Development Policy*. Palgrave Macmillan.

Hoang, Kimberly K. 2013. "Vietnam Rising Dragon: Contesting Dominant Western Masculinities in Ho Chi Minh City's Global Sex Industry." *International Journal of Cultural Sociology* 27: 259–71.

Hoang, Kimberly K. 2014. "Competing Technologies of Embodiment: Pan-Asian Modernity and Third World Dependency in Vietnam's Contemporary Sex Industry." *Gender and Society* 28 (4): 513–36.

Hoang, Kimberly K. 2015. *Dealing in Desire: Asian Ascendancy, Western Decline, and the Hidden Currencies of Global Sex Work*. University of California Press.

Hoang, Kimberly K. 2018. "Risky Investments: How Local and Foreign Investors Finesse Corruption-Rife Emerging Markets." *American Sociological Review* 83 (4): 657–85.

Hoang, Kimberly K., Jessica Cobb, and Ya-Wen Lei. 2017. "Guest Editors' Introduction: Inter-Asian Capital Circulations, Cultural Transformations, and Methodological Positions." *Positions* 25 (4): 633–44.

Hogan, Erica, and Stewart Patrick. 2024. "A Closer Look at the Global South: The Revival of the Concept Signals Enduring Frustration with Inequalities Embedded in the Global Order." Carnegie Endowment for Global Peace. https://carne gieendowment.org/research/2024/05/global-south-colonialism-imperialism? lang=en.

Homei, Aya. 2006. "Birth Attendants in Meiji Japan: The Rise of a Medical Birth Model and a New Division of Labor." *Social History of Medicine* 19 (3): 407–24.

hooks, bell. 1984. *Feminist Theory: From the Margin to the Center*. South End Press.

House Committee on Foreign Affairs. 2022. "China Regional Snapshot: Sub-Saharan Africa." Regional Report. https://foreignaffairs.house.gov/china -regional-snapshot-sub-saharan-africa/.

Htun, Tin Tin. 2013. "Reproductive Rights in Japan: Where Do Women Stand?" In *Critical Issues in Contemporary Japan*, ed. Jeff Kingson, 328. Routledge.

Hu, Shisheng. 2017. "Connecting the 'One Belt and One Road' Initiative with the Interconnected Himalayan Region—Reflections on the Construction of the China-Nepal-India Economic Corridor." In the *Annual Report on the Development of the Indian Ocean Region*, 51–101. Springer.

Hughes, Caroline. 2007. "Transnational Networks, International Organizations and Political Participation in Cambodia: Human Rights, Labour Rights and Common Rights." *Democratization* 14 (5): 834–52.

Hughes, Caroline. 2009. "Dependent Communities: Aid and Politics in Cambodia and East Timor." Cornell University: Southeast Asia Program Publications.

Hughes, Caroline, and Kheang Un, eds. 2011. *Cambodia's Economic Transformation*. Nordic Institute of Asian Studies.

Hunzaker, M. B. Fallin, and Lauren Valentino. 2019. "Mapping Cultural Schemas: From Theory to Method." *American Sociological Review* 84 (5): 950–81.

Hushie, Martin. 2016. "Public-non-governmental Organisation Partnerships for Health: An Exploratory Study with Case Studies from Recent Ghanaian Experience." *BMC Public Health* 16: 963.

Hutchcroft, Paul. 2014. "Linking Capital and the Countryside: Patronage and Clientelism in Japan, Thailand, and the Philippines." In *Clientelism, Social Policy, and the Quality of Democracy*, ed. Diego A. Brun and Larry Diamond, 174–203. Johns Hopkins University Press.

Hwang, Ji-Young, Hi Seap, and Tae-Hee Kim. 2016. "A Comparison of the Cambodian and the South Korean Health Care System." *Journal of Menopausal Medicine* 22 (1): 1–3.

Ichihara, Maiko. 2013. "Understanding Japanese Democracy Assistance." Carnegie Endowment for International Peace. https://carnegieendowment.org/research/2013/03/understanding-japanese-democracy-assistance?lang=en.

ILO (International Labour Organization). 2019. Workers in the Cambodian Informal Economy. Policy Brief. https://www.ilo.org/resource/brief/workers-cambodian-informal-economy.

Indiana Nonprofits Project. 2017. "The Nonprofit Sector in the U.S." https://nonprofit.indiana.edu/our-focus/nonprofit-sector.html#:~:text=Each%20year%20US%20nonprofit%20organizations%20account%20for,11.4Million%20Paid%20Employees.%20*%208.7Billion%20Volunteer%20Hours.

Ingram, George. 2019. "What Every American Should Know about U.S. Foreign Aid." Brookings Institution. https://www.brookings.edu/articles/what-every-american-should-know-about-u-s-foreign-aid/.

Inkenberry, John. 2005. "Power and Liberal Order: America's Postwar World Order in Transition." *International Relations of the Asia-Pacific* 5 (2): 133–52.

Inkenberry, John. 2014. "From Hegemony to the Balance of Power: The Rise of China and American Grand Strategy in East Asia." *International Journal of Korean Unification Studies* 23 (2): 41–63.

Ivaldi, Gilles. 2024. "A Tipping Point for Far-Right Populism in France." In *2024 EP Elections Under the Shadow of Rising Populism*, ed. Gilles Ivaldi and Emilia Zankina. European Center for Populism Studies. https://doi.org/10.55271/rp0070.

Jacobsen, Trude. 2008. *Lost Goddesses: The Denial of Female Power in Cambodian History*. NUS Press.

Jacobsen, Trude. 2008. "Tep Vong, Buddhist Leadership, and Negotiating a 'Middle Path' in Cambodian Politics." In *Profiles in Courage*, ed. Gloria Davies, J. V. D'Cruz, and Nathan Hollier, 129–42. Australian Scholarly Press.

Jacobsen, Trude. 2010. "'Riding a Buffalo to Cross a Muddy Field': Heuristic Approaches to Feminism in Cambodia." In *Women's Movements in Asia: Feminism and Transnational Activism*, ed. Mina Roces and Louise Edwards, 207–23. Routledge.

Jacobsen, Trude. 2011. "Being *broh*: Masculinities in 21st century Cambodia." In *Masculinities in Southeast Asia*, ed. Michele Ford and Lenore Lyons, 86–102. Routledge.

Jacobsen, Trude, and Martin Stuart-Fox. 2013. "Power and Political Culture in Cambodia." *Asia Research Institute*. Working Paper Series No. 200.

Jacques, Claude. 2020. "Ancient Gold in Cambodia." Arts of Southeast Asia. https://artsofsoutheastasia.com/ancient-gold-in-cambodia/.

Jenco, Leigh. 2013. "Revisiting Asian Values." *Journal of the History of Ideas* 74 (2): 237–58.

JICA (Japan International Cooperation Agency). 2005. "Japan's Experiences in Public Health and Medical Systems." https://openjicareport.jica.go.jp/pdf/11868221.pdf.

JICA (Japan International Cooperation Agency). 2005. *Maternal and Child Health Handbook*. https://www.jica.go.jp/Resource/project/angola/001/materials/ku57pq00003sz73v-att/mch_handbook_eng_v3–0.pdf.

JICA (Japan International Cooperation Agency). 2013. "JICA's Operation in the Health Sector: Past and Future." https://www.jica.go.jp/english/our_work/thematic_issues/health/c8h0vm00005zn19g-att/position_paper.pdf.

JICA (Japan International Cooperation Agency). 2016. "What Is Maternal and Child Health Handbook? Technical Brief: Global Promotion of Maternal and Child Health Handbook." https://www.jica.go.jp/english/our_work/thematic_issues/health/c8h0vm0000f7kibw-att/technical_brief_mc_01.pdf.

Johnson, Erik. 2018. "Cambodia Health Equity and Quality Improvement Project (H-EQIP) Gender Assessment." World Bank Document. http://pubdocs.worldbank.org/en/956591524206863227/Cambodia-Health-Equity-and-Quality-Improvement-Project-H-EQIP-Gender-Assessment.

Kamal, Mohd Fairuz Mustaffa, Mohd Salehuddin Mohd Zahari, Mohd Hafiz Hanafiah, and Nurul Wahidah Mohammad Ariffin. 2020. "The Influence of

Japanese Work Cultures on Malaysian Foodservice Employees' Work Stress and Their Turnover Intentions." *Southeast Asian Journal of Management* 14 (2).

Kanji, Nazneen, and Pimbert, Michel. 2003. "Mind the Gap: Mainstreaming Gender and Participation in Development." International Institute for Environment and Development. https://www.iied.org/9259iied.

Kato, Hiroshi. 2013. "Japan's ODA 1954–2014: Changes and Continuities in a Central Instrument in Japan's Foreign Policy." In *The Rise of Development Donors in Asia: Japan's Impact on Emerging Donors*, ed. J. Sato and Y. Shimomura, 11–28. Routledge.

Kato, Shidzue. 1984. *A Fight for Women's Happiness: Pioneering the Family Planning Movement in Japan*. JOICFP Documentary Series 11.

Keck, Margaret E., and Kathryn Sikkink. 1999. *Activists Beyond Borders*. Cornell University Press.

Kentikelenis, Alexandros, and Leonard Seabrooke. 2017. "The Politics of World Polity: Script-Writing in International Organizations." *American Sociological Review* 82 (5): 1065–92.

Kentikelenis, Alexandros, and Thomas Stubbs. 2023. *A Thousand Cuts: Social Protection in the Age of Austerity*. Oxford University Press.

Kermani, Faiz, and Sbita Tia Anna Reandi. 2023. "Exploring the Funding Challenges Faced by Small NGOs: Perspectives from an Organization with Practical Experience of Working in Rural Malawi." *Research and Reports in Tropical Medicine* 14: 99–110.

KFF. 2023. "Breaking Down the U.S. Global Health Budget by Program Area." Global Health Policy. https://www.kff.org/global-health-policy/fact-sheet/breaking-down-the-u-s-global-health-budget-by-program-area/#MCH.

Khazan, Olga. 2020. "The High Cost of Having a Baby in America." *The Atlantic*. https://www.theatlantic.com/health/archive/2020/01/how-much-does-it-cost-have-baby-us/604519/.

Khim, Keovathanak., Laura Goldman, Kristen Shaw, Jeffery Markuns, and Vonthanak Saphonn. 2020. Assessment of Dual Practice Among Physicians in Cambodia. *Human Resources for Health* 18 (1): 18–26.

Kilby, Patrick. 2017. "China and the United States as Aid Donors: Past and Future Trajectories." *Policy Studies and East-West Center* 77. https://www.eastwestcenter.org/publications/china-and-the-united-states-aid-donors-past-and-future-trajectories.

Kim, Hun. 2017. "Capturing World-Class Urbanism Through Modal Governance in Saigon." *Positions: Asia Critique* 25 (4): 669–92.

Klausen, Susanne. 2015. *Abortion Under Apartheid: Nationalism, Sexuality, and Women's Reproductive Rights in South Africa*. Oxford University Press.

Knoema. 2018. "Japan—Maternal Mortality Ratio." World Data Atlas. https://knoema.com/atlas/Japan/Maternal-mortality-ratio.

KOICA (Korean International Cooperation Agency). 2020. Civil Society Cooperation Program. https://www.koica.go.kr/koica_en/3451/subview.do.

Kondoh, Hisahiro, Takaaki Kobayashi, Hiroaki Shiga, and Jin Sato. 2010. "Diversity and Transformation of Aid Patterns in Asia's 'Emerging Donors.'" JICA Research Institute.

Krause, Monika. 2014. *The Good Project: Humanitarian Relief NGOs and the Fragmentation of Reason*. University of Chicago Press.

Kudva, Neema. 2005. "Strong States, Strong NGOs." In *Social Movements in India: Poverty, Power, and Politics*, ed. Raka Ray and Mary Fainsod Katzenstein, 233–66. Rowman and Littlefield Publishers.

Lake, Milli. 2018. *Strong NGOs and Weak States: Pursuing Gender Justice in the Democratic Republic of Congo and South Africa*. Cambridge University Press.

Lamont, Michele, and Virag Molnar. 2002. "The Study of Boundaries in the Social Sciences." *Annual Review of Sociology* 28: 167–95.

Lancaster, Carol. 2007. *Foreign Aid: Diplomacy, Development, Domestic Politics*. University of Chicago Press.

Lange, Thomas. 2020. "Beyond the 'Global' in Global Health Governance: Emerging Health Regionalism and Polycentric Order." SSRN. https://papers.ssrn.com/sol3/papers.cfm?abstract_id=3724332.

Lemay-Herbert, Nicolas, Louis Herns Marcelin, Stephane Pallage, and Toni Cela. 2020. "The Internal Brain Drain: Foreign Aid, Hiring Practices, and International Migration." *Disasters* 44 (4): 621–40.

Levitt, Peggy, and Sally Merry. 2009. "Vernacularization on the Ground: Local Uses of Global Women's Rights in Peru, China, India, and the United States." *Global Networks* 9 (4): 441–61.

Li, Tania. 2005. "Beyond 'the State' and Failed Schemes." *American Anthropologist* 107 (3): 383–94.

Lichterman, Paul, and Nina Eliasoph. 2014. "Civic Action." *American Journal of Sociology* 120 (3): 798–863.

Lilja, Mona. 2016. "(Re)figurations and Situated Bodies: Gendered Shades, Resistance, and Politics in Cambodia." *Signs* 41 (3): 677–99.

Littlejohn, Krystale E. 2021. *Just Get on the Pill*. University of California Press.

Livingston, Gretchen. 2018. "The Changing Profile of Unmarried Parents." Pew Research Center. https://www.pewresearch.org/social-trends/2018/04/25/the-changing-profile-of-unmarried-parents/.

Lu, Michael C., Keisher Highsmith, David de la Cruz, and Hani K. Atrash. 2015. "Putting the 'M' Back in the Maternal and Child Health Bureau: Reducing Maternal Mortality and Morbidity." *Maternal and Child Health Journal* 19:1435–39.

Luker, Kristen. 1985. *Abortion and the Politics of Motherhood*. University of California Press.

Lynch, Caitrin. 2007. *Juki Girls, Good Girls: Gender and Cultural Politics in Sri Lanka's Global Garment Industry*. Cornell University Press.

Mabbett, I. W. 1977. "The 'Indianization' of Southeast Asia: Reflections on the Prehistoric Sources." *Journal of Southeast Asian Studies* 8: 143–61.

Macdonald, Laura. 1995. "A Mixed Blessing: The NGO Boom in Latin America." *NACLA Report on the Americas* 28 (5): 30–35.

Mallik, Rupsa, Eszter Kismodi, and TK Sundari Ravindran. 2023. "The Dynamics of Funding for Sexual and Reproductive Health and Rights (SRHR) Advocacy and Movement Building." *Sexual and Reproductive Health Matters* 31 (3): 1–9.

Mandach, Stefania L., and Georg Blind. 2021. "The Silent Revolution in Japan: Female Labor Market Success from an Aggregate Perspective." In *Corporate Social Responsibility and Gender Equality in Japan*, ed. Gabriel Eweje and Shima Nagano, 159–88. Springer.

Mann, Michael. 2003. *Incoherent Empire*. Verso.

Markovits, David, Austin Strange, and Dustin Tingley. 2019. "Foreign Aid and the Status Quo: Evidence from Pre-Marshall Plan Aid." *Chinese Journal of International Politics* 12 (4): 585–613.

Markowitz, Lisa, and Karen W. Tice. 2002. "Paradoxes of Professionalization: Parallel Dilemmas in Women's Organizations in the Americas." *Gender and Society* 16 (6): 941–58.

Martinsson, Johanna. 2011. "Global Norms: Creation, Diffusion, and Limits." Communication for Governance and Accountability Program (CommGAP) discussion papers. Washington, D.C.: World Bank Group. http://documents .worldbank.org/curated/en/754661468336689726/Global-norms-creation-diffu sion-and-limits.

Matlon, Jordanna. 2022. *A Man Among Other Men: The Crisis of Black Masculinity in Racial Capitalism*. Cornell University Press.

Mawdsley, Emma, Laura Savage, and Sung-Mi Kim. 2014. "A 'Post-Aid World'? Paradigm Shift in Foreign Aid and Development Cooperation at the 2011 Busan High Level Forum." *Geographical Journal* 180 (1): 27–38.

McDonnell, Erin. 2020. *Patchwork Leviathan*. Princeton University Press.

McDonnell, Terence. 2016. *Best Laid Plans: Cultural Entropy and the Unraveling of AIDS Media Campaigns*. University of Chicago Press.

McMichael, Phillip, and Heloise Weber. 2021. *Development and Social Change*. 7th ed. Sage Publications.

Mears, Ashley. 2015. "Working for Free in the VIP: Relational Work and the Production of Consent." *American Sociological Review* 80 (6): 1099–122.

Menon, Alka V. 2023. *Refashioning Race: How Global Cosmetic Surgery Crafts New Beauty Standards*. University of California Press.

Meyer, John W. 2010. "World Society, Institutional Theories, and the Actor." *Annual Review of Sociology* 36: 1–20.

Mies, Maria. 1979. "Towards a Methodology of Women's Studies." *ISS Occasional Papers*. Erasmus University Rotterdam. http://hdl.handle.net/1765/37973.

Miller, Robbi L. 2003. "The Quiet Revolution: Japanese Women Working Around the Law." *Harvard Women's Law Journal* 26: 163–216.

Ministry of Foreign Affairs Japan. 2014. "Japan's 50 Years with OECD." https://www.mofa.go.jp/files/000027193.pdf.

Ministry of Foreign Affairs Japan. 2018. "Opinion Poll on Japan in the African Region." https://www.mofa.go.jp/af/af1/page4e_000790.html.

Ministry of Foreign Affairs Japan. 2022. "TICAD8 Japan's Contribution to Africa." https://www.mofa.go.jp/files/100387226.pdf.

Moghadam, Valentine M. 2005. *Globalizing Women: Transnational Feminist Networks*. Johns Hopkins University Press.

Mohan, Giles, and Kristian Stokke. 2000. Participatory Development and Empowerment: The Dangers of Localism. *Third World Quarterly* 21 (2): 247–68.

Mohanty, Chandra Talpade. 1988. "Under Western Eyes: Feminist Scholarship and Colonial Discourses." *Feminist Review* 30: 65–88.

Mojola, Sanyu A. 2014. *Love, Money, and HIV: Becoming a Modern African Woman in the Age of AIDS*. University of California Press.

Morash, Merry. 2024. *In a Box: Gender-Responsive Reform, Mass Community Supervision, and Neoliberal Policies*. University of California Press.

Morgan, Glen, and Peer Hull Kristensen. 2006. "The Contested Space of Multinationals: Varieties of Institutionalism, Varieties of Capitalism." *Human Relations* 59 (11): 1467–90.

Morgan, Kimberly J,. and Ann Shola Orloff. 2017. *The Many Hands of the State: Theorizing Political Authority and Social Control*. Cambridge University Press.

Mosse, David, and David Lewis. 2006. *Development Brokers and Translators: The Ethnographies of Aid and Agencies*. Kumarian Press.

Mount, Liz. 2024. *"New Women": Trans Women, Hijras, and the Remaking of Inequality in India*. Cambridge University Press.

My, An. 2013. "Childcare Expansion in East Asia: Changing Shape of the Institutional Configurations in Japan and South Korea." *Asian Social Work and Policy Review* 7 (1): 28–43.

Nainar, Ammar. 2024. "India's Foreign Assistance: Trends, Processes, and Priorities." Observer Research Foundation America, Background Paper: Foreign Policy & Security. https://orfamerica.org/newresearch/india-foreign-assistance-priorities.

Nam, Sylvia. 2011. "Phnom Penh: From the Politics of Ruin to the Possibilities of Return." *TDSR* 23 (1): 55–68.

Naples, Nancy A. 2017. "Feminist Methodology." In *The Blackwell Encyclopedia of Sociology*, ed. G. Ritzer. Wiley.

Narayan, Uma. 1997. *Dislocating Cultures/Identities, Traditions, and Third World-Feminism*. Routledge.

Nassanga, Goretti, and Sabiti Makara. 2014. "Perceptions of Chinese Presence in Africa as Reflected in the African Media: Case Study of Uganda." China and Africa Media, Communications and Public Diplomacy.

Nelson, Daniel B., Michelle H. Moniz, and Matthew M. Davis. 2018. "Population-Level Factors Associated with Maternal Mortality in the United States, 1997–2012." *BMC Public Health* 18: 1007.

Neomoto, Kumiko. 2012. "Long Working Hours and the Corporate Gender Divide in Japan." *Gender, Work, and Organization* 20 (5): 512–27.

Nicholls, Samuel T. 2019. "A Moment of Possibility: The Rise and Fall of the New International Economic Order." Master's thesis, University of Adelaide.

Nikles, Brigitte. 2008. "Women, Pregnancy, and Health: Traditional Midwives Among the Bunong in Mondulkiri, Cambodia." *International Survey Network*. Conference Paper. http://www.khmerstudies.org/download-files/publications/Conference_Proceeding/02_part_01_3_BrigitteNikles.pdf?lbisphpreq=1.

Nippon. 2024. "Record 80,000 Female Doctors in Japan, Huge Gender Gap Remains." Japan Data. https://www.nippon.com/en/japan-data/h01978/record-80-000-female-doctors-in-japan-but-huge-gender-gap-remains.html.

Noonan, Rita. 2002. "Gender and the Politics of Needs: Broadening the Scope of Welfare State Provision in Costa Rica." *Gender and Society* 16 (2): 216–39.

Noor, Farhish A. 2021. *The Long Shadow of the 19th Century: Critical Essays on Colonial Orientalism in Southeast Asia*. Matahari Books.

Obeng-Odoom, Franklin. 2024. "China-Africa Relations in The Economist, 2019–2021." *Journal of Asian and African Studies* 59 (3): 1000–1017.

Ochiai, Emiko. 2014. "Leaving the West, Rejoining the East? Gender and Family in Japan's Semi-Compressed Modernity." *International Sociology* 29 (3): 209–28.

OECD (Organisation for Economic Co-operation and Development). 2018. "OECD Development Co-operation Peer Reviews: Korea." https://www.oecd-ilibrary.org/sites/9789264288829-15. en/index.html?itemId=/content/component/9789264288829-15-en.

OECD (Organisation for Economic Co-operation and Development). 2020. "OECD Development Co-operation Peer Reviews: Japan 2020." https://www.oecd.org/en/publications/oecd-development-co-operation-peer-reviews-japan-2020_b2229106-en.html.

OECD (Organisation for Economic Co-operation and Development). 2021. "Development Co-operation Profile: Japan." OECD iLibrary. https://www.oecd-ilibrary.org/sites/b8cf3944-en/index.html?itemId=/content/component/b8cf3944-en.

OECD (Organisation for Economic Co-operation and Development). 2022. "Aid in Support of Gender Equality and Women's Empowerment Donor Charts." OECD Report. https://www.oecd.org/development/financing-sustainable -development/Aid-to-gender-equality-donor-charts-2022.pdf.

Ogasawara, Yuko. 1998. *Office Ladies and Salaried Men: Power, Gender, and Work in Japanese Companies*. University of California Press.

Ojendal, Joakim, and Hans Antlov. 1998. "Asian Values and Its Political Conse-quences: Is Cambodia the First Domino?" *Pacific Review* 11 (4): 525–40.

Okech, Awino, and Dinah Musindarwezo. 2019. "Transnational Feminism and the Post-2015 Development Agenda." *Soundings: A Journal of Politics and Cul-ture* 71: 75–90.

Ong, Aihwa, and Stephen J. Collier. 2007. *Global Assemblages: Technology, Politics, and Ethics as Anthropological Problems*. Blackwell Publishing.

Onzivu, William. 2012. "Regionalism and the Reinvigoration of Global Health Diplomacy: Lessons from Africa." *Asian Journal of WTO and International Health Law and Policy* 7 (1): 49–76.

Open Development Cambodia. 2018. "Aid and Development Report." https:// opendevelopmentcambodia.net/topics/aid-and-development/.

Open Development Cambodia. 2021. "Investment Report." https:// opendevelopmentcambodia.net/topics/investment/.

Osborne, Milton. 1994. *Sihanouk: Prince of Light, Prince of Darkness*. University of Hawaii Press.

Osborne, Stephen P. 2003. *The Voluntary and Non-Profit Sector in Japan*. Rout-ledge.

Otele, Oscar M. 2023. "What Explains African Perceptions of China as a Model of Development?" *Megatrends Afrika*. https://www.swp-berlin.org/assets/afrika /publications/MTA_working_paper/MTA_WP08_2023_Otele_Chinas_ Model_of_Development.pdf.

Packard, Randall M. 2016. *A History of Global Health: Interventions into the Lives of Other Peoples*. Johns Hopkins University Press.

Pal, Kusum Kalo, Saadia Zahidi, and Silja Baller. 2024. "Global Gender Gap Report 2024." World Economic Forum. https://www.weforum.org/publications /global-gender-gap-report-2024/.

Patil, Vrushali. 2022. *Webbed Connectivities: The Imperial Sociology of Sex, Gender, and Sexuality*. University of Minnesota Press.

Pekkanen, Robert. 2000. "Japan's New Politics: The Case of the NPO Law." *Jour-nal of Japanese Studies* 26 (1): 111–48.

Pekkanen, Robert. 2006. *Japan's Dual Civil Society: Members Without Advocates*. Stanford University Press.

Peng, Ito. 2012. "Social and Political Economy of Care in Japan and South Korea." *International Journal of Sociology and Social Policy* 32 (11/12): 636–49.

Petchesky, Rosalind Pollack. 2003. *Global Prescriptions: Gendering Health and Human Rights*. Zed Books.

Petroni, Suzanne, and Patty Skuster. 2008. "The Exportation of Ideology: Reproductive Health and Rights in U.S. Foreign Policy." American Bar Association Report. https://www.americanbar.org/groups/crsj/publications/human_rights _magazine_home/human_rights_vol35_2008/human_rights_winter2008/hr_ winter08_petroni_skuster/.

Pich, Charadine, and Chhengpor Aun. 2023. "How Small States Navigate U.S.-China Rivalry: The Case of Cambodia." Analysis Paper. United States Institute for Peace. https://www.usip.org/publications/2023/09/how-small-states-navi gate-us-china-rivalry-case-cambodia.

Pierotti, Rachel. 2013. "Increasing Rejection of Intimate Partner Violence: Evidence of Global Cultural Diffusion." *American Sociological Review* 78 (2): 240–65.

Pike, Isabel. 2019. "A Discursive Spectrum: The Narrative of Kenya's 'Neglected' Boy Child." *Gender and Society* 34 (2): 284–306.

Plummer, Samantha, Jackie Smith, and Melanie Hughes. 2018. Transnational Human Rights Organizing and Global Health Governance, 1963–2013. *Global Governance* 7 (1): 62–68.

Puri, Joyti. 2003. *Encountering Nationalism*. Wiley-Blackwell.

Puri, Jyoti. 2016. *Sexual States: Governance and the Struggle over the Antisodomy Law in India*. Duke University Press.

Quadagno, Jill. 2010. "Institutions, Interest Groups, and Ideology: An Agenda for the Sociology of Health Care Reform." *Journal of Health and Social Behavior* 51 (2): 125–36.

Radhakrishnan, Smitha. 2011. *Appropriately Indian: Gender and Culture in a New Transnational Class*. Duke University Press.

Radhakrishnan, Smitha. 2022. *Making Women Pay: Microfinance in Urban India*. Duke University Press.

Radhakrishnan, Smitha, and Cinzia D. Solari. 2023. *The Gender Order of Neoliberalism*. Wiley.

Radhakrishnan, Smitha, and Cinzia Solari. 2025. "Beyond #Girlboss and #Tradwife: Reclaiming Joy by Expanding Our Feminist Imagination." *Contexts* 24 (1): 28–33.

Ranabhat, Chhabi, Shambhu Acharya, Chiranjivi Adhikari, and Chun-Bae Kim. 2023. "Universal Health Coverage Evolution, Ongoing Trend, and Future Challenge: A Conceptual and Historical Policy Review." *Frontiers in Public Health* 3 (11).

Rankin, Katharine. 2001. "Governing Development: Neoliberalism, Microcredit, and Rational Economic Woman." *Economy and Society* 30 (1): 18–37.

Ransom, Elizabeth, and Carmen Bain. 2011. "Gendering Agricultural Aid: An

Analysis of Whether International Development Assistance Targets Women and Gender." *Gender and Society* 25 (1): 48–74.

Reed, Steven. 2021. "Patronage and Predominance: How the LDP Maintains Its Hold on Power." *Social Science Japan Journal* 25 (1): 83–100.

Regilme, Salvador Santio. 2023. "United States Foreign Aid and Multilateralism Under the Trump Presidency." *New Global Studies* 17 (1): 45–69.

Reimann, Kim D. 2010. *The Rise of Japanese NGOs: Activism from Above*. Routledge.

Rinaldo, Rachel. 2013. *Mobilizing Piety: Islam and Feminism in Indonesia*. Oxford University Press.

Robinson, Linda. 2023. "Progress on the Status of Women and Girls Off Track in UN Assessment." Council on Foreign Relations. https://www.cfr.org/in-brief/progress-status-women-and-girls-track-un-assessment.

Ros, Bandeth, Gillian Le, Suzanne Fustukian, and Barbara McPake. 2019. "Sociocultural Change in Conflict and Post Conflict Settings: Five Decades of Giving Birth in Cambodia." *Conflict and Health* 13: 53.

Rosenlee, Li-Hsiang. 2023. "Gender in Confucian Philosophy." In *The Stanford Encyclopedia of Philosophy*, ed. Edward N. Zalta and Uri Nodelman. https://plato.stanford.edu/archives/spr2023/entries/confucian-gender/.

Roth, Silke. 2012. "Professionalization Trends and Inequality: Experiences and Practices in Aid Relationships." *Third World Quarterly* 33 (8): 1459–74.

Roth, Silke. 2015. *The Paradoxes of Aid Work: Passionate Professionals*. Routledge.

Said, Edward. 1978. *Orientalism*. Pantheon Books.

Schmitz, Hans Peter, and George E. Mitchell. 2022. "Understanding the Limits of Transnational NGO Power: Forms, Norms, and the Architecture." *International Studies Review* 24 (3): 1–27.

SEEK Development. 2023. "Donor Tracker: South Korea." https://donortracker.org/donor_profiles/south-korea.

Sen, Parama. 2017. "Do Asian Values Still Exist? Revisiting the Roots in Search of a Plausible Future." *South Asian Survey* 21 (1 and 2): 51–63.

Shambaugh, Jay, Ryan Nunn, and Becca Portman. 2017. "Lessons from the Rise in Women's Labor Force Participation in Japan." *Brookings Report*. https://www.brookings.edu/research/lessons-from-the-rise-of-womens-labor-force-participation-in-japan/.

Shih, Elena. 2023. *Manufacturing Freedom: Sex Work, Anti-trafficking Rehab, and the Racial Wages of Rescue*. University of California Press.

Shire, Karen A., and Kumiko Nemoto. 2020. "The Origins and Transformations of Conservative Gender Regimes in Germany and Japan." *Social Politics* 27 (3): 432–48.

Shu, Xialoging, and Jingjing Chen. 2023. *Chinese Marriages in Transition*. Rutgers University Press.

Sibiri, Hagan. 2019. "East Asia in Africa: The 'Rival' Policy Frameworks and the Prospect for Cooperation." *East Asian Community Review* 2: 125–47.

Silver, Laura. 2022. "Populists in Europe—Especially on the Right—Have Increased Their Vote Shares in Recent Elections." Pew Research Center. https://www.pewresearch.org/short-reads/2022/10/06/populists-in-europe-especially-those-on-the-right-have-increased-their-vote-shares-in-recent-elections/.

Singh, Bhubhindar. 2002. "ASEAN's Perceptions of Japan: Change and Continuity." *Asian Survey* 42 (2): 276–96.

Skocpol, Theda, Marshall Ganz, and Ziad Munson. 2000. "A Nation of Organizers: The Institutional Origins of Civic Volunteerism in the United States." *American Political Science Review* 94 (3): 527–46.

Smith, Daniel Jordan. 2003. "Patronage, Per Diems, and the 'Workshop Mentality': The Practices of Family Planning Programs in Southeastern Nigeria." *World Development* 31 (4): 703–15.

Songchuan, Chen, and Chu Shulong. 2011. "Is America Declining?" Brookings Institution. https://www.brookings.edu/opinions/is-america-declining/.

Spires, Anthony. 2012. "US Foundations Boost Chinese Government, Not NGOs." YaleGlobal Online. https://archive-yaleglobal.yale.edu/content/us-foundations-boost-chinese-government-not-ngos.

Stallings, Barbara, and Eun M. Kim. 2017. *Promoting Development: The Political Economy of East Asian Foreign Aid*. Palgrave Macmillan.

Starrs, Ann M. 2006. "Safe Motherhood Initiative: 20 Years and Counting." *The Lancet* 368: 1130–32.

Stevens, Rosemary. 2008. "History and Health Policy in the United States: The Making of the Health Care Industry 1948–2008." *Social History of Medicine* 21 (3): 461–83.

Stroup, Sarah. 2012. *Borders Among Activists: International NGOs in the United States, Britain, and France*. Cornell University Press.

Suh, Siri. 2021. *Dying to Count: Post-Abortion Care and Global Reproductive Health Politics in Senegal*. Rutgers University Press.

Swidler, Ann. 1986. "Culture in Action: Symbols and Strategies." *American Sociological Review* 51 (2): 273–86.

Swidler, Ann, and Susan Cotts Watkins. 2017. *A Fraught Embrace: The Romance and Reality of AIDS Altruism in Africa*. Princeton University Press.

Swiss, Liam. 2018. *The Globalization of Foreign Aid*. Routledge.

Takegawa, Shogo. 2009. "International Circumstances as Factors in Building a Welfare State: Welfare Regimes in Europe, Japan and Korea." *International Journal of Japanese Sociology* 18 (1): 79–96.

Takeuchi, Jiro, Yu Sakagami, and Romana Perez. 2016. "The Mother and Child Health Handbook in Japan as a Health Promotion Tool: An Overview of Its

History, Contents, Use, Benefits, and Global Influence." *Global Pediatric Health* 3: 1–9.

Taniguchi, Rie, and Sarah Babb. 2009. "The Global Construction of Development Models: The U.S., Japan, and the East Asian Miracle." *Socio-Economic Review* 7 (2): 277–303.

Tarnoff, Curt, and Marian L. Lawson. 2016. "Foreign Aid: An Introduction to U.S. Programs and Policy." In Congressional Research Service 7 5700 R40213. US Congress.

Tavory, Iddo, and Ann Swidler. 2009. "Condom Semiotics: Meaning and Condom Use in Rural Malawi." *American Sociological Review* 74 (2): 171–89.

Taylor, Charles. 2004. *Modern Social Imaginaries*. Duke University Press.

Thayer, Mille. 2010. "Translations and Refusals: Re-signifying Meanings as Feminist Political Practice." *Feminist Studies* 36 (1): 200–230.

Thomas, Mandy. 2004. "East Asian Cultural Traces in Post-Socialist Vietnam." In *Rouge Flows: TransAsian Cultural Traffic*, ed. Koichi Iwabuch, Stephen Muecke, and Mandy Thomas, 177–96. Hong Kong University Press.

Thornton, Arland, Shawn F. Dorius, and Jeffery Swindle. 2015. "Developmental Idealism: The Cultural Foundations of World Development Programs." *Sociology of Development* 1 (2): 69–112.

Thul, Prak Chan. 2017. "Defiant Hun Sen Tells U.S. to Cut All Aid to Cambodia." *Reuters*. https://www.reuters.com/article/us-cambodia-usa/defiant-hun-sen-tells-u-s-to-cut-all-aid-to-cambodia-idUSKBN1DJ049.

Tonami, Aki. 2018. Exporting the Developmental State: Japan's Economic Diplomacy in the Arctic. *Third World Quarterly* 39 (6): 1211–25.

Trends. 2024. "Foreign Direct Investment in Africa: Trends and Prospects." Trends: Economic Studies Section. https://trendsresearch.org/insight/foreign-direct-investment-in-africa-trends-and-prospects/.

Tripp, Aili Mari. 2006. "The Evolution of Transnational Feminisms: Consensus, Conflict, and New Dynamics." In *Global Feminisms: Transnational Women's Activism, Organizing, and Human Rights*, ed. Myra Marx Ferree and Aili Mari Tripp, chap. 3. NYU Press.

Tsing, Anna. 2021. *The Mushroom at the End of the World: On the Possibility of Life in Capitalist Ruins*. Princeton University Press.

Tsutsui, Kiyoteru. 2018. *Rights Make Might: Global Human Rights and Minority Social Movements in Japan*. Oxford University Press.

Turshen, Meredith. 2020. *Women's Health Movements: A Global Force for Change*. Palgrave Macmillan.

Un, Kheang. 2005. "Patronage Politics and Hybrid Democracy: Political Change in Cambodia 1993–2003." *Asian Perspectives*, 29 (2): 203–230.

UN (United Nations). 2020. "Conferences on Women and Gender Equality." https://www.un.org/en/conferences/women/beijing1995.

UNCTAD (United Nations Conference on Trade and Development). 2020. "World Investment Report: Country Fact Sheet Cambodia." https://unctad .org/system/files/non-official-document/wir20_fs_kh_en.pdf.

United Nations Cambodia. 2020. "Gender Equality Deep-Dive for Cambodia." Common Country Analysis. https://cambodia.un.org/sites/default/files/2022 -03/Gender%20Deep%20Dive%20-%20CCA%20Cambodia_V6_010322_LQ .pdf.

UN Women (United Nations Women). 2023. "1 in Every 10 Women in the World Lives in Extreme Poverty." https://www.unwomen.org/en/news-stories/press-re lease/2024/03/1-in-every-10-women-in-the-world-lives-in-extreme-poverty.

USAID (United States Agency for International Development). 2012. "Gender Equality and Women's Empowerment Policy." https://www.usaid.gov/sites/ default/files/documents/1865/GenderEqualityPolicy_0.pdf.

USAID (United States Agency for International Development). 2014. "Ending Preventable Maternal Mortality: USAID Maternal Health Vision for Action." https://www.usaid.gov/sites/default/files/documents/1864/MCHVisionOne Pager_0.pdf.

USAID (United States Agency for International Development). 2016. "Gender Analysis Cambodia." USAID, Phnom Penh, Cambodia.

U.S. Bureau of Labor Statistics. 2019. Press Release: Employment Characteristics of Families—2019. https://www.bls.gov/news.release/archives/famee_04212020 .pdf.

U.S. Department of Health and Human Services. 2012. TANF Financial Data. Office of Family Assistance. https://acf.gov/ofa/data/tanf-financial-data-fy-2012.

U.S. Department of State. 2025. "U.S. Relations with Vietnam." https://www.state .gov/u-s-relations-with-vietnam/.

Valle, Firuzeh Shokooh. 2023. *In Defense of Solidarity and Pleasure: Feminist Tech-nopolitics in the Global South*. Stanford University Press.

Vandenberg-Daves, Jodi. 2014. *Modern Motherhood: An American History*. Rutgers University Press.

Vicheika, Kann. 2023. "Reflection: 30 Years of Women in Cambodian Politics." *Heinrich Böll Stiftung*. https://www.boell.de/en/2023/12/20/reflection-30-years -women-cambodian-politics.

Vijayakumar, Gowri. 2021. *At Risk: Indian Sexual Politics and the Global AIDS Crisis*. Stanford University Press.

Vong, Streytouch, Bandeth Ros, Rosemary Morgan, and Sally Theobald. 2019. "Why Are Fewer Women Rising to the Top? A Life History Gender Analysis of Cambodia's Health Workforce." *BMC Health Services Research* 19: 595.

Viterna, Jocelyn, Emily Clough, and Killian Clarke. 2015. "Reclaiming the 'Third Sector' from 'Civil Society': A New Agenda for Development Studies." *Sociology of Development* 1 (1): 173–207.

Walby, Sylvia. 2020. "Varieties of Gender Regimes." *Social Politics* 27 (3): 414–31.

Welsh, Bridget, and Alex Chang. 2015. "Choosing China: Public Perceptions of China as a Model." *Journal of Contemporary China* 24 (93): 442–56.

White, Alexandre I. R. 2023. *Epidemic Orientalism: Race, Capital, and the Governance of Infectious Disease.* Stanford University Press.

Whitley, Richard D. 1991. "The Social Construction of Business Systems in East Asia." *Organizational Studies* 12 (1): 1–28.

WHO (World Health Organization). 2016. "Cambodia-WHO Country Cooperation Strategy 2016–2020." WHO Western Pacific. https://www.who.int/publications/i/item/WPRO-2016-DPM-004.

Wike, Richard, Bruce Stokes, Jacob Poushter, and Russ Oates. 2014. "Global Opposition to U.S. Surveillance and Drones, But Limited Harm to Americans' Image." Pew Research Center. https://www.pewresearch.org/wp-content/uploads/sites/20/2014/07/2014-07-14-Balance-of-Power.pdf.

Wilks, Mary-Collier. 2019. "Activist, Entrepreneur, or Caretaker? Negotiating Varieties of Women in Development." *Gender and Society* 33 (2): 224–50.

Wilks, Mary-Collier. 2021. "Embodying Feminism: Donor Demands and Bridgework in Cambodian Nongovernmental Organizations." *Gender, Work and Organization* 29 (2): 575–90.

Wilks, Mary-Collier, Derek Richardson, and Jennifer Bair. 2021. "International NGOs in Global Aid Chains: Linking Donors, Local Partners, and the State." *Sociology of Development* 7 (1): 1–24.

Woods, Ngaire. 2008. "Whose Aid? Whose Influence? China, Emerging Donors and the Silent Revolution in Development Assistance." *International Affairs* 84 (6): 1205–21.

World Bank. 2018. "Government Effectiveness." GovData360. https://govdata360.worldbank.org/indicators/h580f9aa5?country=KHM&indicator=388&countries=USA,JPN&viz=line_chart&years=1996,2018.

Worley, Will. 2024. "International Aid Agencies Pay the Price for Boom and Bust." *New Humanitarian.* https://www.thenewhumanitarian.org/analysis/2024/08/29/international-aid-agencies-pay-price-boom-and-bust.

Wyrod, Robert. 2008. "Between Women's Rights and Men's Authority: Masculinity and Shifting Discourses of Gender Difference in Urban Uganda." *Gender and Society* 22 (6): 799–823.

Wyrod, Robert. 2019. "In the General's Valley: China, Africa, and the Limits of Developmental Pragmatism." *Sociology of Development* 5 (2): 174–97.

Yamashita, Junko. 2012. "Citizen Participation or Low-Cost Care Providers? Welfare Non-Profit Organizations in Japan." *Social Science Japan Journal* 16 (1): 45–62.

Yoshida, Honami, Haruka Sakamoto, Auska Leslie, Osamu Takahashi, Tsuboi

Satoshi, and Kunio Kitamura. 2016. "Contraception in Japan: Current Trends." *Contraception* 93 (6): 475–77.

Zhang, Chuanhong, and Zhenqian Huang. 2023. "Foreign Aid, Norm Diffusion, and Local Support for Gender Equality: Comparing Evidence from the World Bank and China's Aid Projects in Africa." *Studies in Comparative International Development* 58: 584–615.

Zelizer, Viviana. 2012. "How I Became a Relational Economic Sociologist and What Does That Mean?" *Politics and Society* 40 (2): 145–75.

Zippel, Kathrin. 2006. *The Politics of Sexual Harassment*. Cambridge University Press.

Index

Note: Page numbers in italics indicate figures. Numbers in bold indicate tables.

For a complete listing of titles in this series, visit the
Stanford University Press website, www.sup.org.

The authorized representative in the EU for product safety and compliance is:
Mare Nostrum Group
B.V Doelen 72
4831 GR Breda
The Netherlands

www.ingramcontent.com/pod-product-compliance
Lightning Source LLC
Chambersburg PA
CBHW020852270326
41928CB00006B/671